Advances in Anatomy, Embryology and Cell Biology
Ergebnisse der Anatomie und Entwicklungsgeschichte
Revues d'anatomie et de morphologie expérimentale

51/2

Editors
A. Brodal, Oslo · W. Hild, Galveston · J. van Limborgh, Amsterdam
R. Ortmann, Köln · T. H. Schiebler, Würzburg · G. Töndury, Zürich · E. Wolff, Paris

A. Raedler, J. Sievers

Influences of Experimental Brain Edema on the Development of the Visual System

With 27 Figures

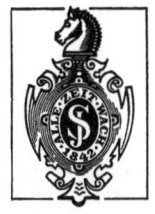

Springer-Verlag Berlin Heidelberg New York 1975

Dr. Andreas Raedler and Dr. Jobst Sievers
Anatomisches Institut der Universität Hamburg
2000 Hamburg 20, Martinistraße 52
Federal Republic of Germany

Library of Congress Cataloging in Publication Data. Raedler, A., 1947—Influences of experimental brain edema on the development of the visual system. (Advances in anatomy, embryology and cell biology; v. 51/2). Bibliography: p. Includes index. 1. Cerebral edema. 2. Embryology, Experimental. 3. Pathology, Experimental. 4. Developmental neurology. I. Sievers, Jost, 1948—joint author. II. Title. III. Series. [DNLM: 1. Brain edema—Chemically induced. 2. Retina—Growth and development. 3. Visual cortex—Growth and development. 4. Visual pathways—Growth and development. W1 AD433K v. 51 fasc. 2 / WW101 R134i]. QL801.E67 vol. 51, fasc. 2 [RB125] 574.4'08s 75-4852 ISBN 978-3-540-07205-8 (Springer-Verlag, New York) [599'.3233]

ISBN 978-3-540-07205-8   ISBN 978-3-642-66092-4 (eBook)
DOI 10.1007/978-3-642-66092-4

Contents

Introduction

The experimental brain edema as a result of application of numerous different toxic agents has been the subject of a large number of publications (for synopses see Hirano, 1969; Long et al., 1965). A concept that took the underlying causes of the lesions as the basis for classification of different types of brain edema was presented by Klatzo (1967). In this classification Klatzo differentiates between cytogenic and vasogenic causes of brain edema that are distinguishable from each other by the differing behaviour and reaction of the blood-brain-barrier. The vasogenic type of brain edema is found mostly in the vicinity of tumors, traumata and foci of infections, presumably because of an alteration of the conditions of permeability, as well as in brain edemas that are caused by changes in the hemodynamics of the central nervous system, and toxic substances that act directly on the wall of the blood vessel. The cytogenic type of brain edema in many experimental models is the result of, for instance, TET-intoxication, water intoxication, poisoning with other chemical substances and anoxia. Its direct cause according to Klatzo (1967) is to be seen in a disturbance of the intracellular osmoregulation of the parenchymal cells. Although the composition of the edema fluid is dependent on the type of toxic substance used, the lack of plasma proteins in the edema fluid is characteristic for the brain edemas of this group.

The sensibility of the different cells of the immature brain against various toxic agents has been studied by a limited number of authors only. Especially noticeable are the studies of Hicks (1955, 1958, Hicks et al., (1959, 1962), and Hicks and d'Amato (1961), in which conclusions about specializations of the metabolism of differentiating cells could be drawn from the effects of the administration of different noxae. Wolfe et al. (1962) observed alterations of various glia cells in addition to lesions in motor neurons of the anterior horn of the spinal cord after treatment of young postnatal rats with the antimetabolite 6-aminonicotinamide (6-AN).

Streicher et al. (1965) compared the effects of application of cold and TET on immature and adult brains of rats and cats. In the case of application of cold they observed a definitely higher resistance of the immature brains against edema formation, after TET-intoxication on the other hand they found that the qualitative damages differed only slightly. In further investigations Fleischhauer and Schmalbach (1968) reported that a different edematous and cytological reaction was induced in the immature brain according to the date of intracerebral injection of aluminium hydroxide before or after myelination. Before the formation of myelin sheaths they neither found a brain edema nor a gliosis, both of which appeared very pronouncedly after completion of myelination. Similar differences of reaction of the immature brain after application of traumatic noxae, which had already been described by von Gudden (1840) and Spatz (1921), were confirmed electron microscopically by Sumi and Hager (1968a, b). Cowen *et al.* (1970) described the temporal sequence and the types of lesion and their healing after treating the cerebral cortices of young rats with repeated electric shocks.

The object of this study is to demonstrate the different types of reaction of the individual nerve and glia cell precursors in various phases of development and specific regions of the central nervous system to the application of a brain edema-producing agent—in this case 6-aminonicotinamide. Both the morphological alterations and the detailed knowledge of the pharmacological mechanism of action of 6-AN should allow to draw conclusions about the importance of the interrelation of nerve cells and neuroglia for the development of the neuropil, the blood-brain-barrier, the functional and nutritional unit neuron-glia as well as the histological lamination of specific neural structures.

Material and Methods

Rat embryos of day 11 through 21 of gestation and postnatal rats of 0, 1, 2, 3, 5, 7, 10 and 14 days of age were used as material for this study. The exact time of gestation was determined with the following method: Wistar albino rats were kept in temperature and humidity-controlled cages in a shifted day-night-rhythm. After mating between 7.30 and 9.30 a.m. the successful copulation was controlled by a vaginal smear for sperms. The day of demonstration of sperms was taken as day 0. On day 22 of gestation the young rats were born.

The individual experimental groups consisted of 3 pregnant rats, from each of which four embryos were taken for further investigation. The pregnant rats were injected with 8 mg/kg body weight of 6-AN, the postnatal young rats with 10 mg/kg body weight.

Table 1 shows the experimental set-up of injection and sacrifice of the rat embryos and postnatal young rats.

Table 1

	10	12	16	18	19	20	0	2	5	7	Date of treatment
11	0										
12	0										
13		0									
14	0	0									
16	0	0									
18	0	0									
19				0							
20				0	0						
21	0	0		0	0	0					
0											
1							0				
2							0				
3							0				
5							0				
7							0				
10							0				
14							0	0	0	0	
Date of sacrifice											

Fixation. The brain of the rat embryos were fixed by immersion in a solution of 6% glutaraldehyde in a 0.05 mol phosphate buffer. The postnatal young rats were supravitally perfused with the same fixing solution. Later in the course of our experiments a perfusion technique for embryos was developed and by comparison with these controls we were able to confirm the cytological alterations induced by 6-AN as such and not as artefacts caused by fixation by immersion.

Preparation of the Brain. Embryos of 11 days of age were processed for electron microscopy in toto, from the brains of 13, 14 and 15 days old fetuses cross sections of less than 1 mm thickness through the mesencephalon and the prosencephalon as well as both eyes were taken for further processing. Beginning on day 16 of gestation the regions corresponding to the optic centers of the diencephalon, mesencephalon, and the cerebral cortex were cut out of the whole brain. Again tissue pieces of about 1 mm thickness and of an area corresponding to the respective brain stem or cortical level were prepared and taken for both light and electron microscopic investigation. The eyes were either divided at the level of the optic nerve or, in later stages of gestation and postnatally were cut into a kind of a ring at the level of the nervus opticus. Especially the tissue pieces obtained from the postnatal animals by this method of preparation had quite large dimensions, a satisfactory postfixation with osmium tetroxide, however, was guaranteed by the thinness of the specimens.

The tissue pieces obtained by this method of preparation were postfixed in a 1% OsO_4 solution in a 0.1 mol phosphate buffer including 0.1 mol saccharose for 2 hours at 4° C, dehydrated in ethanol of increasing concentrations and embedded in Epon 812 (Luft, 1961).

Embedding. The embedding of the tissue pieces was modified in the following way. After initial polymerization at 37° C for about 10–12 hours the tissue pieces are taken out of the very viscous Epon, which is allowed to drip off, enclosed with a thin, flexible plastic foil and then further polymerized at the temperatures recommended by Luft (1961). The polymerized tissue block then is covered by a very thin film of Epon only, which makes obsolete the trimming procedure of the Epon blocks that is necessary after conventional embedment of the tissue specimens in gelatine capsules or small plastic boxes, and facilitates obtaining the most superficial tissue sections which are fixed best, at optimal orientation of the surface of the tissue block. Moreover, foldings of tissue sections, that especially occur when semi-thin sections of structures with large lumina like the retina and the embryonal cerebral cortex and brain stem are placed on glass-slides are completely absent.

Semithin sections of the whole material were made on a Reichert OMU 2 ultramicrotome and stained with a 5 to 2 mixture of Janus green and Darrow Red (Sievers, 1971). Photographic montages at 225-fold enlargement through the whole width of the four optic centers were made in order to better follow the cytological and laminary development of the neural structures studied. Regions typical of and important for the development of the individual optic centers were selected from these montages and the tissue blocks were then trimmed correspondingly for electron microscopy. Ultra-thin sections were cut on glass and diamond knives on Reichert OMU2 and Porter ultramicrotomes, contrasted with uranyl acetate and lead citrate (Reynolds, 1961) and studied and photographed with a Siemens Elmiskop I.

Notes on Terminology. The terminology mostly used in neuroembryology is based in its fundamental aspects on His's (1889, 1894) concept of two different cell populations in the embryonal central nervous system, the germinal cells which produce the neuroblasts, and the spongioblasts, which serve both as a syncytial framework and produce the glioblasts. The neural wall is then subdivided into the germinal layer, the mantle layer that consists of neuroblasts, and the cell sparse marginal layer. The denotation of these layers was often changed in the light of new findings for instance of pathological or autoradiographic nature. In order to replace the often confusing terminology by a sensible, uniform nomenclature that takes into consideration the recent cytophotometric, autoradiographic and electron microscopic findings, a committee of mostly American neuroscientists constituted itself at Boulder, Colorado, USA in 1969. In the committee report it is suggested to denominate the layers fundamental to the development of the brain according to geotopographical criteria and thus subdivide the neural wall into a ventricular, a subventricular, an intermediate and a marginal zone. The neuroblast layer that in the development of the cerebral and cerebellar cortices appears at the junction of the intermediate and marginal zones is named the cortical plate. The cells of the different layers have corresponding denotations like ventricular and subventricular cells. These give rise to future nerve cells as well as to glioblasts that later according to certain features may be subdivided into astroblasts and oligodendroblasts. This new terminology

8

devised by the Boulder Committee was accepted and used in our study. A further problem of nomenclature in neurogenesis was also discussed at Boulder, the term neuroblast, which implicates a generative potency of a cell that in reality is postmitotic. The dilemma of this term was considered yet the discussion did not lead to the formulation of a new cell name. We propose to name as preneurons postmitotic neural cells in the brain wall which are in a specific interval of development, between the stage of beginning ramification and the stage of orientation of ergastoplasm that will be explained in the discussion of this study.

Results

Treatment on Day 10 of Gestation

Sacrifice on Day 11 of Gestation

The cerebral cortex of the embryos treated on day 10 and sacrificed on day 11 of pregnancy is thinner compared to that of control animals. Its inner limiting border has a very irregular shape caused by lumpy protrusions in some sites and marked recesses in others. The lumpy protrusions which were also found in other brain regions and on other days of treatment, appeared ultrastructurally as cytoplasmic protrusions of the inner processes of the ventricular cells lacking organelles. Neither the protrusions and the processes nor the perikarya of the ventricular cells exhibit ultrastructural alterations. These findings are valid not only for the cerebral cortex but in the same way for the brain stem too.

Sacrifice on Day 14 of Gestation

Four days after treatment practically all ventricular cells in the cerebral cortex display large optically empty spaces of up to nuclear size that mostly have an oval to round shape and usually seem to be directly connected with the nucleus. These large spaces in the electron microscope appear as voluminous swellings of the perinuclear space and in some cases also of the cytoplasmic granular endoplasmic reticulum. The former will henceforth be termed perinuclear cisterns. Moreover pyknotic nuclei, macrophages and extravasated erythrocytes which mainly lie in small clusters among the ventricular cells, are found scattered throughout the whole neural wall. Regions with a very marked hemorrhagic component show comparatively little spongy alterations.

The extent of these pathological alterations seems to be correlated to the thickness of the cortical wall, for in the thin dorsal part of the cerebral cortex that has a thickness of only a few rows of cells and is not yet vascularized, only slight or no alterations were found. A comparable spongy appearance with additional pyknoses, macrophages and extravasations of erythrocytes was observed in the brain stem and—with the exception of the last component—in the retina as well.

Sacrifice between Days 15 and 21 of Gestation

The development of and reactions to these pathological lesions could not continually be followed since the rate of resorption of the embryos treated at such an early date in development reached approximately 100%. We obtained two litters of embryos on day 21 of gestation which also exhibited an extremely large rate of resorption. The histological investigation of these animals showed a nearly complete compensation of all pathological alterations in the regions studied, which, however, seemed slightly hypoplastic. It can therefore not be excluded

9

that the fetuses studied on day 21 of gestation either exhibited a smaller sensitivity to the intoxicating agent or that they were not exposed to the damaging noxa to the same degree as the other animals.

Treatment on Day 12 of Gestation

Sacrifice on Days 13 and 14 of Gestation

Retina. On day 13 of pregnancy the beginning vacuolization or swelling of the ventricular cells was observed (Fig. 2). This process is advanced—at least focally—in the pigment epithelium, where single cells exhibit not only a large perinuclear cistern but also massive swellings of the granular endoplasmic reticulum in their cytoplasm.

One day later the whole ventricular zone of the retina is affected by a profound swelling of its cells which exhibits a gradient of alteration that increases towards the inner aspects of the retina. The processes of the ventricular cells at the outer margin of the retina show the same cytoplasmic protrusions into the former optic ventricle as those of the cerebral cortex and the brain stem one day p.i. on day 10 of gestation. The most severe alterations appear in the pigment epithelium which is markedly widened by the extreme ballooning of the perinuclear cisterns and the other membrane systems of the cytoplasm as well as the intercellular spaces.

Sacrifice on Days 13 and 14 of Gestation

Brain Stem. The ventricular cells of the brain stem contain large swollen perinuclear cisterns in their perikarya both on the 13th and 14th days of gestation (Fig. 1), that impress as detachments of the outer nuclear membrane with characteristic flattening of the nucleus at the site of their largest diameter. Within these cisterns loops consisting of single membranes are often found without recognizable continuity with the membrane limiting the perinuclear cistern. The granular endoplasmic reticulum is also dilated in many places of the perikaryon, often reaching into the primitive processes. The perikarya of other cells seem to be filled with sharply delimited vacuoles that are surrounded by very little cytoplasm and cannot definitely be associated with other cell organelles. The nucleus and the outer nuclear membrane are not altered. These cells resemble the "gitter cells" that more often appear postnatally.

On the 14th day of gestation the hydrops of the ventricular cells is enlarged further. However, the appearance of the alterations is also characterized by numerous pyknoses that are scattered throughout the neural wall and leave out

Fig. 1. Mesencephalon of a rat fetus on embryonal day 13, 24 hours after application of 6-AN. Hydropic alteration of the whole neural wall mostly in the form of perinuclear cisterns. × 760

Fig. 2. Fetal rat retina on day 14 after application of 6-AN on embryonal day 12. The alterations in the nervous part of the retina correspond to those of the brain stem and the cerebral cortex. The pigment epithelium is more severely affected since the intracellular vacuolar dilatation is not restricted to the perinuclear cleft but all membrane-bound spaces in the perikaryal cytoplasm are swollen. × 288

Fig. 3. Brain stem of a rat fetus on embryonal day 14, 48 hours after treatment with 6-AN. Massive extravasations of erythrocytes are found in the neural wall which spare only the region in the direct vicinity of the ventricle. The tissue appears less edematously altered,

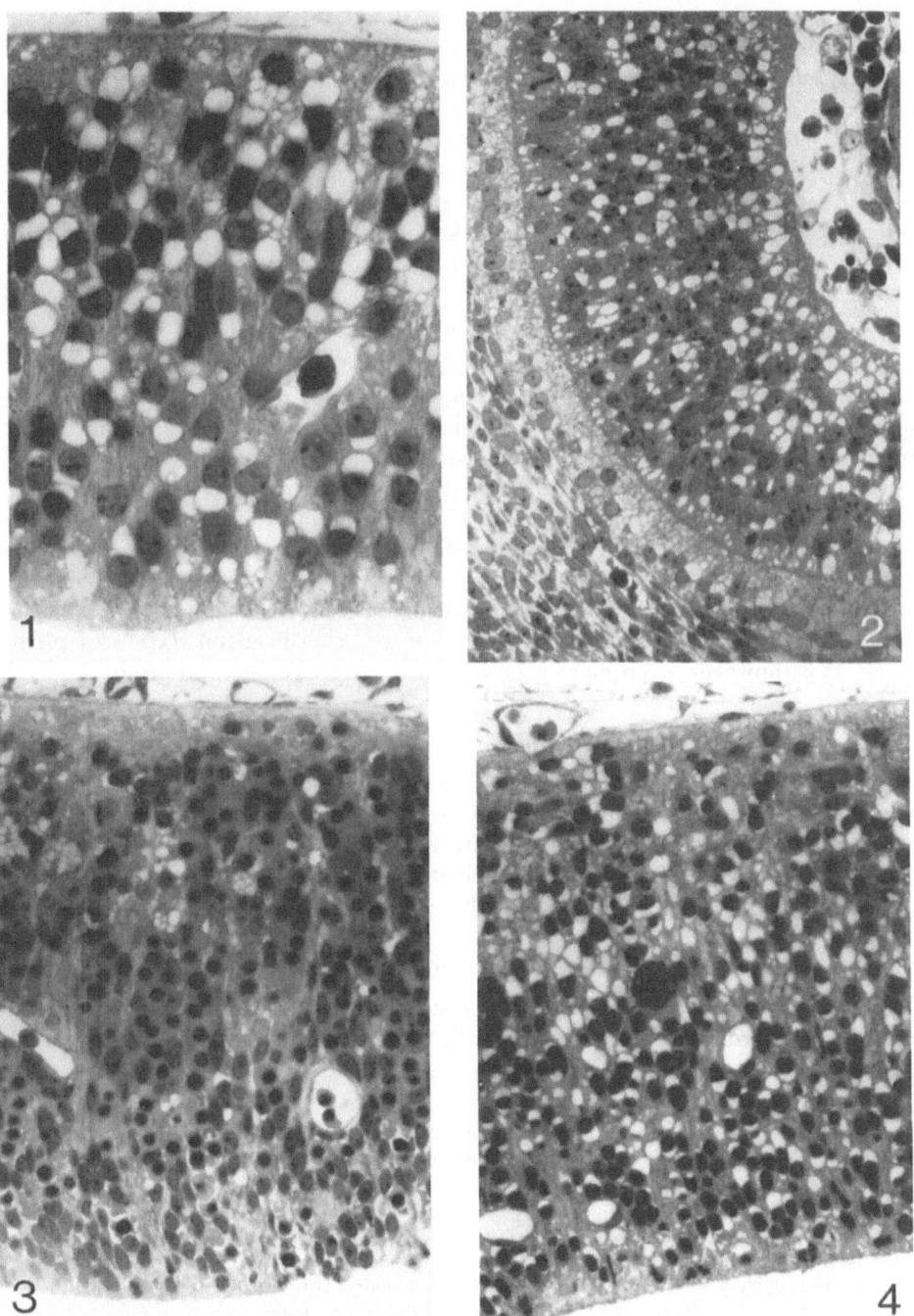

especially the perinuclear cisterns that usually are the most frequent pathological lesions are very rare. Instead small vesicular foci are found among the rows of erythrocytes. × 288

Fig. 4. Occipital cortex of a rat fetus on embryonal day 14, 48 hours after treatment with 6-AN. Hydropic alteration of the neural wall, near the ventricle mostly in the form of perinuclear cisterns, in the marginal zone as small vesicular swollen processes. Macrophages and free erythrocytes are seen in the edematously altered tissue. × 288

only the outermost zones, as well as extravasations of erythrocytes (Fig. 3) in well defined locations where the swelling of the ventricular cells is less marked. In the marginal zone vacuoles are also found, which may be associated with the rough endoplasmic reticulum in the outer processes of the ventricular cells. The results of these lesions are numerous indentations of the ventricular wall and a general asymmetry of the brain stem. The differentiating preneurons lying mainly in small clusters between the fiber bundles that appear in the intermediate zone of the mesencephalon on day 14 of gestation, and that are characterized by rounder and lighther nuclei are not affected by the hydropic alterations.

Sacrifice on Days 13 and 14 of Gestation

Cortex cerebralis. Two days after application of 8 mg 6-AN/kg body weight severe swellings of the ventricular cells characterized by detachments of the outer from the inner nuclear membrane and small to bullous dilatations of the scarce endoplasmic reticulum of these cells are observed besides a slight hypoplasia of the whole cerebral cortex and irregular indentations of the neural wall (Fig. 4). The rest of the cell organelles, e.g. mitochondria and Golgi complexes, are well preserved and demonstrable. At the inner margin of the cortical wall the inner processes of the ventricular cells protrude beyond the inner limiting membrane of desmosomes into the ventricle, a finding that already has been described for the embryos treated on day 10 and sacrificed on day 11 of pregnancy. It is, however, even more pronounced in this experimental group.

Sacrifice on Day 16 of Gestation

Retina. In the retina the swelling of the cells of the ventricular zone has been largely reduced and is now limited essentially to the inner and central parts of the retina as well as the cells of the pigment epithelium (Fig. 5). The differentiated cells at the inner margin of the ventricular zone appear to be diminished in number in comparison to control animals.

Sacrifice on Day 16 of Gestation

Brain Stem. Similar findings may be observed in the superior colliculus where most of the hydropic cells are limited to the outer part of the ventricular zone and

Fig. 5. Retina of a rat fetus on embryonal day 16 after application of 6-AN on day 12 of pregnancy. Cytoplasmic dilatations and pyknotic alterations in the pigment epithelium. In the nervous part of the retina the edema is more pronounced in the inner (older) section. × 510

Fig. 6. Mesencephalon of a rat fetus on day 16 of gestation four days after treatment with 6-AN on embryonal day 12. The edematous alterations as well as the macrophages and extravasated erythrocytes very characteristically are concentrated in the middle third of the brain wall. Macrophages are also found in the ventricular lumen. × 192

Fig. 7. Retina of a rat fetus on day 20 of gestation after treatment with 6-AN on embryonal day 12. Marked formation of folds of the nervous part of the retina that reach up to the lens. While the proliferative part of the retina, the ventricular zone, retains a constant width within the folds, the ganglion cell layer above the folds is thinly attenuated and pyknotic. In the stalk of the folds a homogeneous, grey precipitate is seen between the two corresponding limiting membranes. The ganglion cell layer and the ventricular zone are spongily altered, whereby perinuclear cisterns predominate in the latter. The pigment

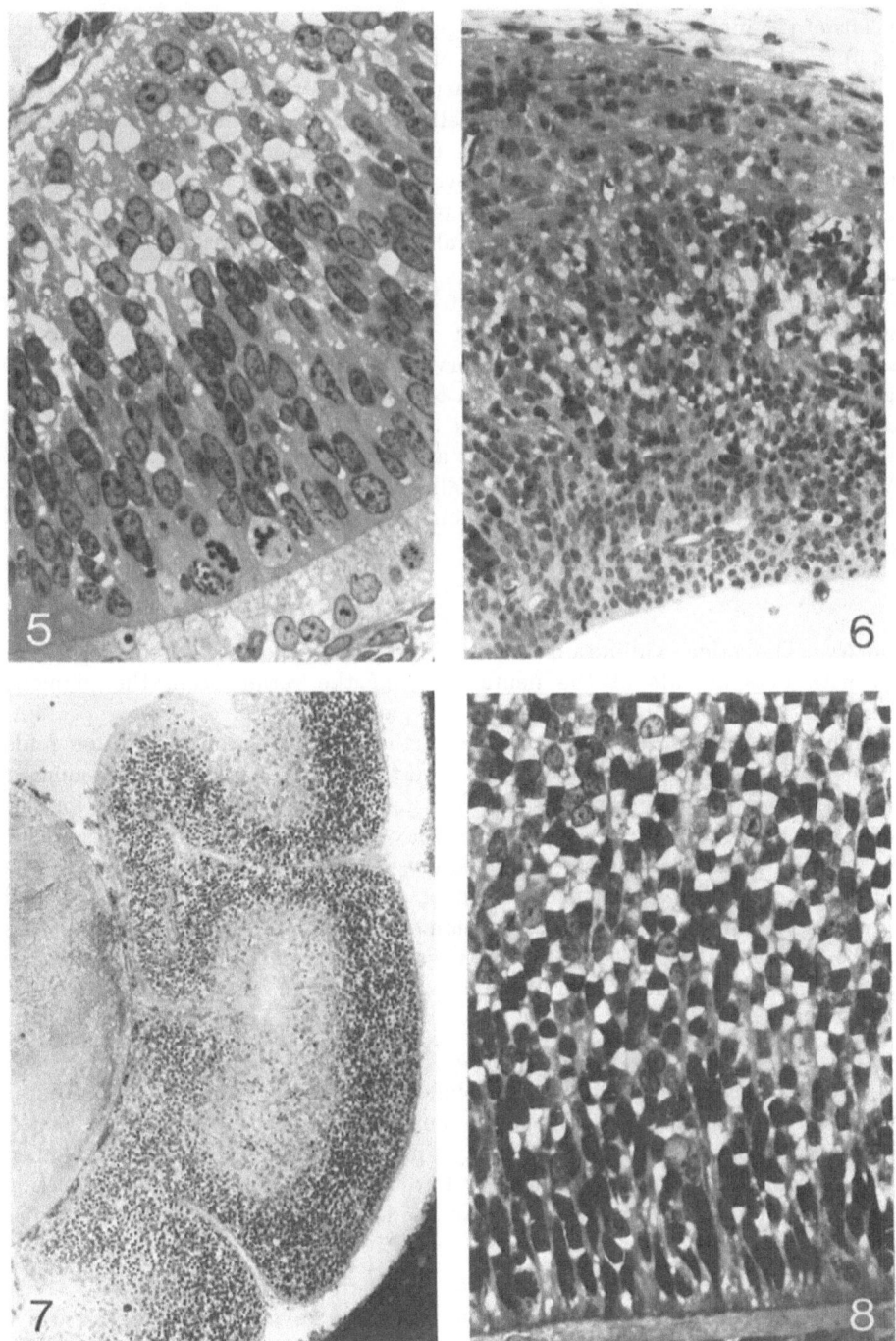

epithelium exhibits comparatively few lesions. Pyknoses are found in all layers. The cleft between the pigment epithelium and ventricular zone is artificial, dependent on the homogeneous substance between both cell layers that has decreased their cohesion. × 75

Fig. 8. Ventricular zone of the rat retina one day after birth, 24 hours after application of 6-AN. Severe edema of the retinal ventricular zone in the form of swollen perinuclear cisterns. × 480

the cells of the intermediate zone that migrate towards the outer collicular layers (Fig. 6). In the median proliferation zone of the superior colliculi that appears on the 16th or 17th day of gestation (see Raedler and Sievers, 1974) and represents a locus of proliferation, spongily altered cells are totally absent. Besides scattered pyknoses and extravasated erythrocytes numerous macrophages are especially noticeable. In the embryonic stages of development the latter are also present in untreated animals, mostly in regions with tendencies to regression, e.g. the lamina terminalis in the telencephalon and central positions of the retina near the optic stalk.

The ultrastructural characteristics of these cells will be described below. Moreover, large cells with dark yet not pyknotic nuclei and numerous cytoplasmic vacuoles ("gitter cells") were observed. These may not only be demonstrated in the neural tissue but also within the ventricular lumen or seemingly on their way to that site.

In the diencephalon the pathological alterations following intoxication with 6-AN have regressed further than in the colliculus superior, it remains a retardation of the diencephalic development for about one day as well as a quite severe disorder in its histological structure.

Sacrifice on Day 18 of Gestation

Retina. The retina exhibits a pronounced formation of folds that reach up to the lens, with detachments of the neural part of the retina from the pigment epithelium, the space between these two parts being filled with a proteincontaining precipitate. While the width of the ventricular zone in these folds remains unchanged the ganglion cell layer and the nerve fiber layer are attenuated over the protruding ventricular cells. In some animals focal extravasations of erythrocytes were found in the ganglion cell layer. The majority of the ventricular cells which is edematously altered for the most part exhibits perinuclear cisterns and round, optically empty spaces often of nuclear size. Among them—as well as in the ganglion cell layer and the pigment epithelium—numerous pyknoses may be recognized. In spite of the pyknoses and the cytoplasmic swellings the pigment epithelium is less severely altered than the nervous part of the retina.

Sacrifice on Day 18 of Gestation

Brain Stem. Neither in the mesencephalon nor in the diencephalon of the rat embryos of embryonal day 18 are permanent alterations of either the cells or the histological structure recognizable 6 days p.i. The brain stem centers studied exhibit a retardation of development of 1 to $1^1/_2$ days. The retarded maturation of the colliculus superior usually refers to the as yet unformed definitive regular lamination.

Sacrifice on Day 18 of Gestation

Cortex cerebralis. On the 18th embryonal day (6 days p.i.) usually the width of the bipolar cortical plate and the intermediate zone is reduced in the cerebral cortex, the number of fiber bundles in the subventricular and intermediate zones is drastically diminished. The cytological differentiation on the other hand does not appear to be disturbed. The lag in development which in comparison to control animals amounts to $1-1^1/_2$ days has not fully been compensated even on day 21 of gestation.

14

Treatment on Day 16 of Gestation

Sacrifice on Days 18 and 21 of Gestation

Retina. All layers of the retina including the pigment epithelium exhibit the typical spongy alterations. Affected most are the inner zone of the ventricular layer and the inner plexiform layer that is just beginning to differentiate. The cells of the pigment epithelium display a vacuolization of their cytoplasm by swollen endoplasmic reticulum besides the enlargement of the perinuclear space, while in the ventricular cells the intracellular edema is mainly limited to the perinuclear cistern. Within the cisterns the free loops that have been described above already, are often seen. In the presumptive ganglion cell layer, too, numerous dilatated spaces are recognizable, which, however, must be associated with the inner processes of the ventricular cells in the outer part of the retina, if one is not to postulate that the processes of the ganglion cells react to the intoxicating agent in a manner different from their perikarya.

In the perikarya of the ganglion cells neither a detachment of the outer from the inner nuclear membrane nor a dilatation of the endoplasmic reticulum is seen. In all retinal layers, especially in the inner plexiform layer and the inner portion of the ventricular zone, pyknotic nuclei as well as macrophages are demonstrable.

On day 21 of pregnancy the retina—in the same way as the group treated on day 12—is very much folded exhibiting the characteristics described above, e.g. constant width of the ventricular zone with concomitant pronounced attenuation of the ganglion cell layer over the foldings of the ventricular zone, which are contacting the overlying lens because of the extremely hypoplastic vitreous body. All layers are severely pyknotic. Within the folds or between ventricular zone and pigment epithelium protein-like precipitates are observed.

Sacrifice on Days 18 and 21 of Gestation

Brain Stem. The smallest alterations are found in the brain stem in the form of usually moderate swellings of the perinuclear space of the subventricular cells and some pyknoses in this region. On day 21 of gestation this intracellular edema has regressed and the brain stem appears normal in its histological structure.

Sacrifice on Days 18 and 21 of Gestation

Cortex cerebralis. The ventricular cells and some of the cells in the intermediate zone are affected by the intracellular edematous alterations in the form of perinuclear cisterns, while the cells in the bipolar cortical plate and the differentiating preneurons in the definite layers of the cerebral cortex in the multipolar part of the cortical plate appear totally intact.

The ventricular cells bordering the ventricle display the cytoplasmic protrusions of their inner processes and the contractions of the neural wall that already has been described above and that could be the result of intensive focal proliferations or uncompensated well defined necroses. As only consequences of these acute damages pyknoses of ventricular cells are found on day 21 of gestation. All other alterations have regressed and the cerebral cortex appears hypoplastic in spite of a normal histological structure.

Treatment on Day 18 of Gestation

Sacrifice on Days 19, 20 and 21 of Gestation

Retina. In the outer layers of the ventricular zone a typical intracellular hydrops begins to appear in the ventricular cells one day p.i. In a few, closely defined sites, the start of a detachment of the ventricular zone from the pigment epithelium is seen (Fig. 7). The intermediate space appears to be filled with a structured, protein-like precipitate. This morphological alteration may possibly represent the initial step in the formation of retinal folds, which on day 20 of gestation have grown for quite some distance and partly reach up to the lens. The inner space of these folds is also filled with the protein-like material described above. Above the folds, the ganglion cell layer is maximally attenuated; it retains its normal width only between the folds. All cells with the exception of the ganglion cells and the differentiated cells at the inner margin of the ventricular zone are more or less edematously altered.

The increased number of pyknoses and macrophages in the inner part of the ventricular zone indicates the distribution of the damaged undifferentiated cells which is reduced from the inside of the retina toward its outside during the continual proliferation of the ventricular cells.

Sacrifice on Days 19, 20 and 21 of Gestation

Brain Stem. The alterations on days 19 and 20 of gestation in the brain stem are limited to a transient edematous reaction of the subventricular cells or other as yet undifferentiated cells which has already been compensated 3 days p.i.

Sacrifice on Days 19, 20 and 21 of Gestation

Cortex cerebralis. The reaction to the intoxication with 6-AN as in the brain stem of earlier days becomes progressively less intense in the cerebral cortex. The typical hydropic alterations and pyknoses of the ventricular cells as well as of most of the undifferentiated cells in the subventricular and intermediate zones are observed. The cells of both the bipolar and the multipolar parts of the cortical plate are not altered at all.

Treatment on Day 19 of Gestation

Sacrifice on Days 20 and 21 of Gestation

Retina. In the retina the formation of folds with corresponding edematous and pyknotic alterations is again found, however, the extent of damage seen in the animals treated on day 12 or 16 of pregnancy is not reached.

Sacrifice on Days 20 and 21 of Gestation

Brain Stem, Cortex cerebralis. In the brain stem and cerebral cortex the ventricular cells and most of the undifferentiated cells in the subventricular and intermediate zones exhibit a slight spongy alteration. Overall the reaction of this group does not differ significantly from that of the animals treated on day 18 and 19 of pregnancy.

Treatment on the Day of Birth

Sacrifice on the First Postnatal Day

Retina. Light microscopic alterations of the pigment epithelium consist essentially of vacuolar swellings of the cytoplasm, ultrastructurally they appear as numerous swollen membrane-bound profiles that often can be identified as dilated granular endoplasmic reticulum by the closely-packed ribosomes on their membranes. The mitochondria are well preserved, the Golgi complexes not swollen. The intercellular clefts of the pigment epithelium are maximally dilated and can be distinguished from the other vacuolar spaces only with difficulty. The damage of the pigment epithelium is distinctly focal so that significant regional differences exist.

In the ventricular zone especially the outer part is severely damaged (Fig. 8). The light microscopical round vacuoles near the nucleus are electron microscopically recognizable as perinuclear cisterns between the inner and outer nuclear membranes, often containing an inner loop, and markedly swollen granular endoplasmic reticulum (Fig. 9).

The Golgi complexes of the ventricular cells are not swollen, or only minimally dilated. The differentiated cells of the ganglion cell layer are not changed even ultrastructurally. In the cytoplasmic structures and processes that surround the differentiated cells of the ventricular zone as well as the ganglion cells, swollen optically empty spaces are likewise found.

Sacrifice on the First Postnatal Day

Brain Stem. Light microscopically, alterations cannot be seen in the structures of the brain stem studied. Electron microscopically some preneurons exhibit finger-like evaginations of the outer nuclear membrane and dilatations of the subsurface cisterns. Most of the glioblasts do not show any kind of reaction, some react with a beginning detachment of the outer nuclear membrane and a swelling of the granular endoplasmic reticulum (Fig. 12), which partly contain free inner loops.

Sacrifice on the First Postnatal Day

Cortex cerebralis. The cerebral cortex also does not exhibit significant light microscopically visible alterations. The ultrastructural findings correspond to those in the brain stem.

Sacrifice on the Second Postnatal Day

Retina. The pigment epithelium still exhibits the regionally differing severe vacuolization of its cells. The ventricular zone has developed a gradient of damage that is directed from the outside of the retina to the inside (Fig. 10), the ventricular cells directly below the differentiated cells at the inner margin of the ventricular zone being damaged most. They are characterized by the typically flattened nuclear pole at the base of the large perinuclear cistern. In this zone of the most severe injury macrophages are accumulated while pyknoses are uniformly distributed throughout all retinal layers. The differentiated cells at the inner margin of the ventricular zone as well as in the ganglion cell layer appear undamaged. Large vacuoles have been formed in the inner plexiform and also in the nerve fiber layer. In the central portions of the retina an additional cell layer

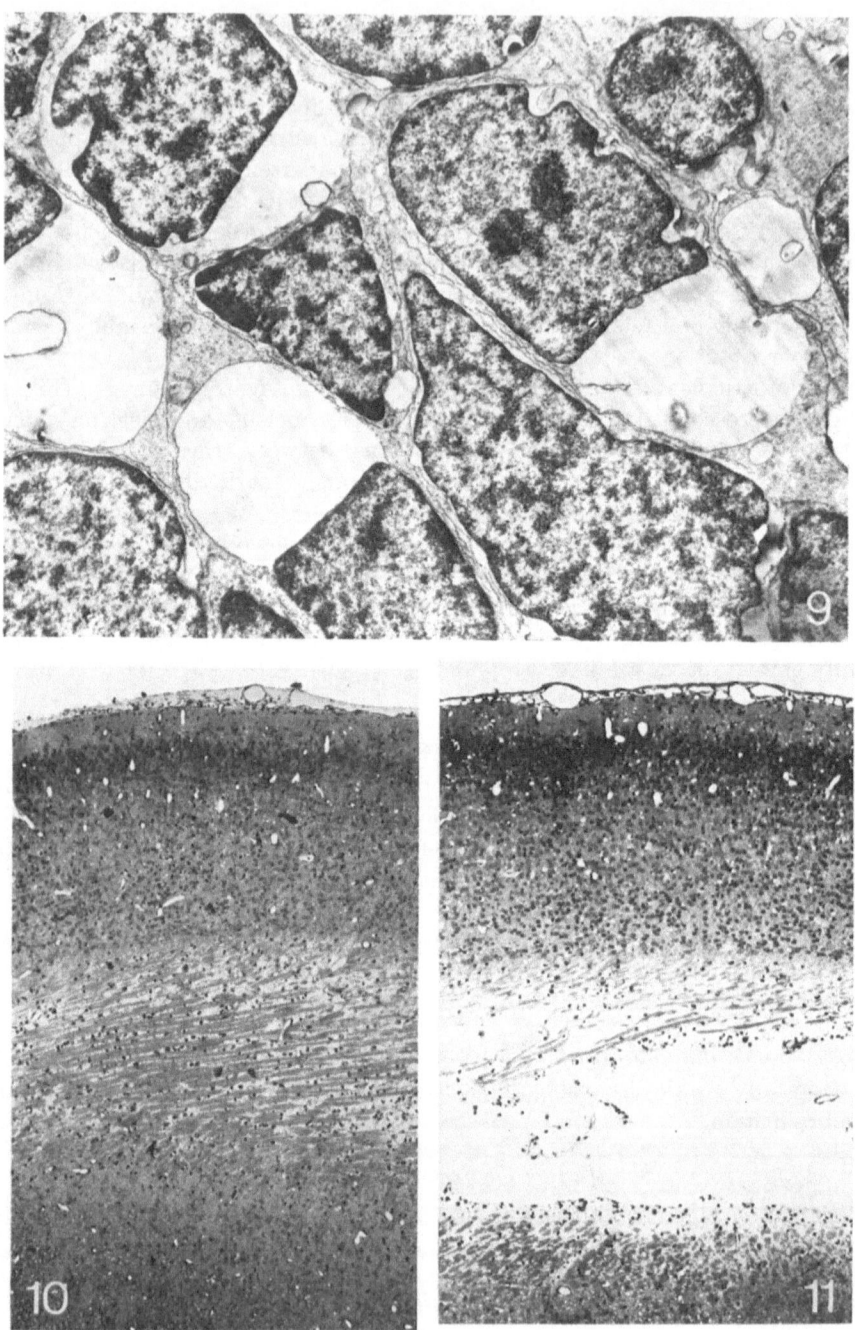

Fig. 9. Ventricular cells of the rat retina one day after birth, 24 hours after treatment with 6-AN. Perinuclear cisterns of the ventricular cells with severe deformations (flattening) of their nuclei. Within the swollen spaces free inner loops are often found. × 6000

Fig. 10. Frontal section of the occipital cortex of the rat three days after birth and application of 6-AN. Diminution of the number of fibers in the cerebral medulla. Rounded glia cells and scattered macrophages are situated between the individual fibers. Large extracellular spaces are lying between the fiber bundles. × 56

is beginning to be formed within the inner plexiform layer. The majority of its cells have the same differentiated appearance as the cells at the inner margin of the ventricular zone. Some undifferentiated cells of this new layer are altered by vacuolar distensions in their cytoplasm.

Sacrifice on the Second Postnatal Day

Brain stem. The alterations do not significantly differ from those described for the first postnatal day. The changes in the preneurons seem to have regressed, for they were not observed 2 days p.i.

Sacrifice on the Second Postnatal Day

Cortex cerebralis. Light microscopically small, optically empty vacuoles, single or in clusters, often in relation to a nucleus are seen in all layers of the cerebral cortex including the fiber layer beneath the cortical grey. In the latter, large extracellular spaces appear between individual fibers and fiber bundles. The different glioblastic cells between the fibers have also changed their structure and shape, some have become rounded, others have enlarged by the formation of numerous small vacuoles in their round perikarya. Electron microscopically a distinct swelling of the granular endoplasmic reticulum of many glioblasts both in their perikarya and processes is found, most of all in the cortical grey matter.

Sacrifice on the Third Postnatal Day

Retina. The distinct gradient of cytological damage that is increasing from the outside toward the inside of the retina, as well as the additional cell layer in the inner plexiform layer have become much more pronounced.

Sacrifice on the Third Postnatal Day

Corpus geniculatum laterale. The opening of the glia chambers of Held can be observed beginning in some vessels. In the perikarya and processes of the later glia cells small vacuolar dilatations have been formed, which are found much more frequently in the cell bodies than in their distended processes at the vessels. Pyknoses are distributed uniformly over the whole lateral geniculate body.

Sacrifice on the Third Postnatal Day

Colliculus superior. In the superior colliculi, too, the glia chambers of Held begin to open and the number of vacuolar swellings of processes in the neuropil increases. Pyknoses also are uniformly distributed throughout all collicular layers. In the perikaryal cytoplasm of many glioblasts a foamy vesicular structure has been formed by the distension of the endoplasmic reticulum (Fig. 14). The damage of the presumptive glia cells is most pronounced near the ventricle and decreases towards the pial basement membrane.

Fig. 11. Rat occipital cortex five days after birth and treatment with 6-AN. The alterations in the cerebral grey correspond to those described on the third postnatal day. In the cerebral medulla the attenuation of fibers has progressed further. The glioblasts seem to form a more or less complete chain or border against the empty innermost space. × 56

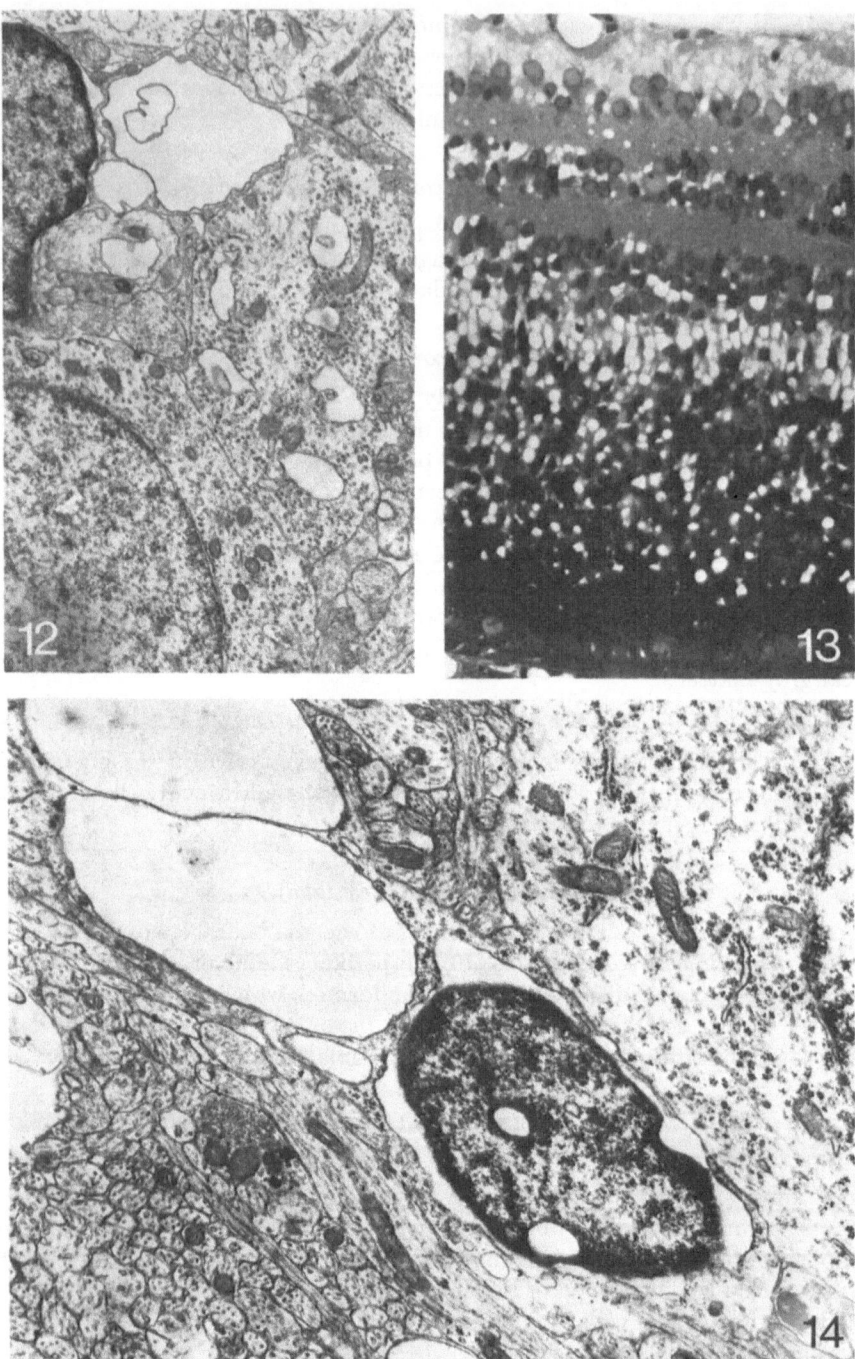

Fig. 12. Different cells of the corpus geniculatum laterale of the rat one day after birth (treatment with 6-AN 24 hours before). Early reaction of the glioblasts in the form of a slight dilatation of the perinuclear cleft and the endoplasmic reticulum. × 9000

Fig. 13. Rat retina five days after birth and treatment with 6-AN. The situation in the pigment epithelium, the ventricular zone, and the ganglion cell layer corresponds to that on the third postnatal day. Remarkable is the formation of an additional nuclear layer in the

Sacrifice on the Third Postnatal Day

Cortex cerebralis. In the processes and perikarya of the small dark polymorphous cells of the molecular layer cytoplasmic vacuoles and perinuclear cisterns appear. These same cytological changes are observed only sporadically in the bipolar cortical plate, while in the deeper layers of the definite cortex, the multipolar cortical plate, vacuoles are more often present both in the neuropil and in the cytoplasm of small undifferentiated cells. Between the axonal fiber bundles in the future white matter that have been attenuated and further pushed apart by enlarging extracellular spaces even more gitter cells and glioblasts enlarged by perinuclear cisterns are found which often lie within the very large extracellular spaces. At numerous vessels the glia chambers of Held are opening up, which, contrary to later stages, have not yet as many individual chambers. Pyknoses are observed in all cortical layers.

Electron microscopically the perikarya of the bipolar cortical plate and the differentiating preneurons of the deeper definite cortical layers do not exhibit cytological alterations. The light microscopical vacuolar alterations in this zone consist of the known distensions of the granular endoplasmic reticulum in glioblasts. In the deepest layers of the definite cerebral cortex both damaged and intact glia cell precursors are found.

In the zone of attenuation of the axonal fibers the young axons pass in small bundles through a large empty space. Between them numerous small cells are localized the nuclei of which resemble those of undifferentiated glioblasts and which have a remarkably thin perikaryon with long slender processes. Within the perikarya and/or the processes of a large part of these cells the system of endoplasmic reticulum is distended giving them the light microscopical appearance of gitter cells.

Some damaged processes exhibit small round vesicles with a dark grey matrix that could suggest either synaptic vesicles or swollen microtubules.

Sacrifice on the Fifth Postnatal Day

Retina. In the pigment epithelium the same situation of focal damage to its cells exists. In the ventricular zone too, the alterations have not decisively been changed; more accentuated is the zone of maximal injury below the differentiated cells of this layer (Fig. 13). The cells at the inner margin of the ventricular zone as well as the cells of the additional cell layer within the inner plexiform layer have become further differentiated and have attained almost the same state of development as the ganglion cells. The sporadic undifferentiated cells of this new layer contain the perinuclear cisterns and vacuoles typical

inner plexiform layer between ventricular zone and ganglion cell layer, and the further enlargement of the swollen processes in the nerve fiber layer. Besides the differentiated cells undifferentiated cells with swollen perinuclear cisterns are found in the ganglion cell layer, the newly formed layer and the inner part of the ventricular zone. × 256

Fig. 14. Glioblast of the rat colliculus superior three days after birth and treatment with 6-AN. The membrane systems of the glioblasts, especially the perinuclear cleft and the endoplasmic reticulum are severely dilatated. The perinuclear cisterns often invaginate digitally into the nuclei of the cells. These invaginations on cross sections appear like intranuclear vacuoles. The cytoplasm of the cells is thinly drawn out around the large vacuoles. × 12000

21

for a 6-AN-intoxication. In the nerve fiber layer as well as the inner plexiform layer numerous processes are severely swollen. The division of the ventricular zone into inner and outer nuclear layers by the differentiating horizontal cells contrary to the control group has not yet taken place. Pyknoses are found in all retinal layers. In the region of the future ora serrata the damage of the retina has reached its maximum. Here the whole ventricular zone has disintegrated as a consequence of the destruction of the injured ventricular cells.

Electron microscopically it is seen that the pigment epithelial cells that light microscopically appeared intact are also affected by the intoxication with 6-AN. The apical portion of these cells is not bordered by long, slender finger-like cytoplasmic protrusions. These seem to have been flattened. In the cytoplasm of the pigment epithelial cells numerous small, densely-packed milky vacuoles are observed, but only a few propigment granules. The other cell organelles seem to be unaltered. The corresponding photoreceptor processes show slight retardation of their development compared to those of control animals. The cytoplasm of the severely affected cells of the pigment epithelium is filled with enormously large vacuoles. In the wedges between these vacuoles small patches of cytoplasm containing ribosomes and mitochondria are localized. The vacuoles are irregularly delimited and in their lumina often exhibit membranes in the form of inner loops. The short thin cytoplasmic processes of the pigment epithelial cells into the intercellular clefts and the communicating basal extracellular space are levelled off like the apical cytoplasmic processes. The photoreceptor processes corresponding to these severely damaged cells are elongated, attenuated and bent parallel to the external limiting membrane.

Many of the cells at the outer margin of the ventricular zone show the typical reactions to an intoxication with 6-AN: perinuclear cisterns and distended profiles of ergastoplasm. In the inner parts of this layer these swellings reach up to nuclear size. The nuclei of the damaged cells in their nucleoplasm exhibit light, round vacuoles which presumably are formed by finger-like invaginations of the inner nuclear membrane into the inner part of the nucleus. Between these extremely ballooned spaces thinly attenuated cytoplasm or just naked membranes are situated. In the differentiated part of the ventricular zone and in the additional cell layer in the inner plexiform layer preneurons with light nuclei and polarized cytoplasm containing abundant ergastoplasm which display no or only minimal pathological alterations, as well as a few other undifferentiated severely damaged cells are observed between maximally distended processes. In the nerve fiber layer likewise very numerous swollen processes are present which may unambiguously be identified as primitive processes of the ventricular cells.

The endfeet of the Müller and ventricular cells at the inner basement membrane at least in part are interspersed with often indistinctly delimited vacuoles. The endothelial cells in the vessels of the nerve fiber layer apparently are not altered.

Sacrifice on the Fifth Postnatal Day

Corpus geniculatum laterale. As in the colliculus superior of the preceding days, in the diencephalon, too, a distinct gradient of damage that decreases from the ventricle toward the pial basement membrane is observed. Specifically in the corpus geniculatum laterale, the distribution and density of the intracytoplasmic distensions and perinuclear cisterns in the small, dark glioblasts correspond to that in the superficial grey of the cerebral cortex. The other findings are well comparable to those of the superior colliculus. Electron microscopically a swelling of all membrane systems is observed in the glioblasts whereby the cytoplasm is maximally attenuated toward the periphery of the cells. The cytoplasm of some preneurons contains small, membrane-bound, optically empty spaces, that cannot be definitely associated with characteristic cell organelles. This finding which can also be observed in other brain parts is present especially often in the vicinity of maximally damaged glioblasts.

Sacrifice on the Fifth Postnatal Day

Colliculus superior. The alterations at the vessels in the form of open glia chambers of Held, in the neuropil, and in the perikarya of glia cell precursors have progressed. In the median zone of proliferation of the superior colliculus especially the small polymorphous cells exhibit the characteristic swellings of their perinuclear cisterns, while the fibers that pass vertically towards the median sulcus of the colliculi superiores are markedly vacuolated (Fig. 27).

The presumptive ependyma is totally disintegrated, partly destroyed. The glia chambers of Held have enlarged. The superficial collicular zones remain relatively unaffected by the cytological alterations, only directly beneath the pial basement membrane many of the constituent processes are markedly distended and foamily altered. In the whole collicular region pyknoses are found. The ultrastructural findings are comparable to those in the lateral geniculate body.

Sacrifice on the Fifth Postnatal Day

Cortex cerebralis. In the grey matter of the cerebral cortex the cytological lesions have become more pronounced: enlargement of Held's glia chambers, increased appearance of partly univesicular, partly multivesicular vacuoles, and additional pyknoses. The fiber bundles in the white matter have been attenuated even further (Fig. 11). Freely between them, in the extremely large extracellular spaces, lie rounded glia cell precursors, "gitter cells", small vessels, pyknoses and different macrophages. In the remaining patches of connected glioblasts numerous mitoses take place. In some glioblasts, presumably oligodendroblasts, that extend their processes through the empty extracellular spaces and that have rounded their perikarya, pathological alterations cannot be seen even ultrastructurally. This also applies to the preneurons and young neurons of the deep cortical layers. Other cells, which in some aspects resemble astroblasts display a widely distended perinuclear cistern and their processes that reach up to the vessels of the fiber layer, are extremely dilatated and separated from the partly disintegrated vascular basement membrane. Thus the extracellular space between the basement membrane and the astroblastic processes becomes distended at many sites of the vessels and in other places the endothelial cells of the vessels come into direct contact with the system of intercellular spaces of the cerebral wall.

In still other glioblasts numerous highly active, large Golgi complexes are seen to have appeared. Many of the glia cell precursors in the presumptive white matter cannot definitely be categorized, for they exhibit ultrastructural criteria common to both glioblasts, gitter cells, and other macrophages.

Sacrifice on the Seventh Postnatal Day

Retina. The swelling of the pigment epithelium has partly regressed, in the ventricular zone the differentiation of the outer plexiform layer by the formation of the horizontal processes of the horizontal cells is seen to begin, clearly separating an outer zone with relatively few vacuoles and perinuclear cisterns from an inner zone with very numerous perinuclear cisterns and complicatedly structured vacuolar complexes. The horizontal cells themselves do not appear to be altered. The nerve fiber layer is severely swollen, however, between the distended processes of the ventricular and Müller cells bundles of intact optic fibers are found. Perinuclear cisterns in the ganglion cell layer, the additional cell layer, and the inner margin of the inner nuclear layer are always associated with small, dark undifferentiated cells.

Sacrifice on the Seventh Postnatal Day

Corpus geniculatum laterale. The situation in the lateral geniculate body is comparable to that on the third postnatal day. In the pedunculi cerebri which contain the efferent cortical fibers large vacuoles are seen; they have somewhat regressed in density in comparison to the fifth postnatal day. The thickness of the pedunculi cerebri is further reduced in comparison to control animals than in preceding stages.

Electron microscopically the preneurons appear intact. Only in preneurons in the vicinity of severely damaged glioblasts a discrete swelling of the granular endoplasmic reticulum is recognizable, in the same manner as in the superior colliculus and cerebral cortex. The glioblasts on the other hand exhibit a marked swelling of their granular endoplasmic reticulum especially in those processes that surround the brain vessels. In this case a thin lamella of cytoplasm is situated directly at the vessel, it is followed by the optically empty space of the extremely distended process and the opposite thin rim of cytoplasm or membrane. In some regions the extracellular space between the vascular processes has become enlarged by the formation of a so-called pseudo-extracellular space through the rupturing of cell membranes of the processes.

Sacrifice on the Seventh Postnatal Day

Colliculus superior. The gradient of damage from the ventricular zone towards the pial basement membrane described above, becomes even more distinct in this stage of the pathological reaction by a further increase of the sequences of the intoxication. The vacuoles have become even larger and often multivesicular, pyknoses are increasingly found in all collicular layers. The glia chambers of Held and the extracellular space next to the vessels are further dilatated. The perikaryal alterations of the glioblasts are more pronounced. In some places the membranes of the severely distended processes are ruptured. The superficial collicular layers again are relatively uninjured.

Fig. 15. Glioblast of the occipital cortex of the rat seven days after birth and treatment with 6-AN. Detachment of the outer nuclear membrane and formation of a markedly distended perinuclear cistern. Between the glioblastic perikaryon and the vascular basement membrane (left part of the photograph) intact processes are situated. × 10000

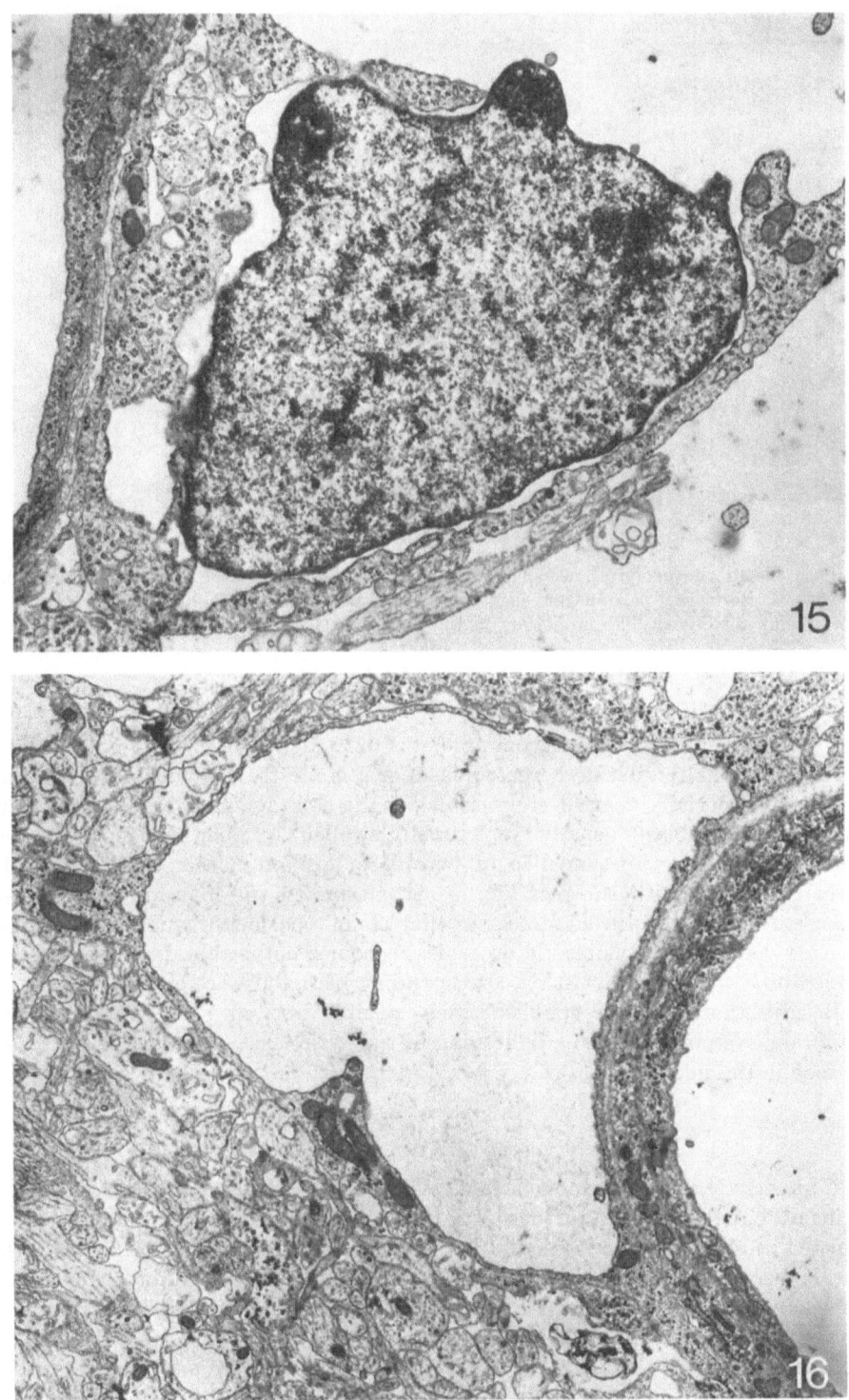

Fig. 16. Vessel in the occipital cortex of the rat seven days after birth and treatment with 6-AN. Dilatation of an astroblastic process (glia chamber of Held) × 8000

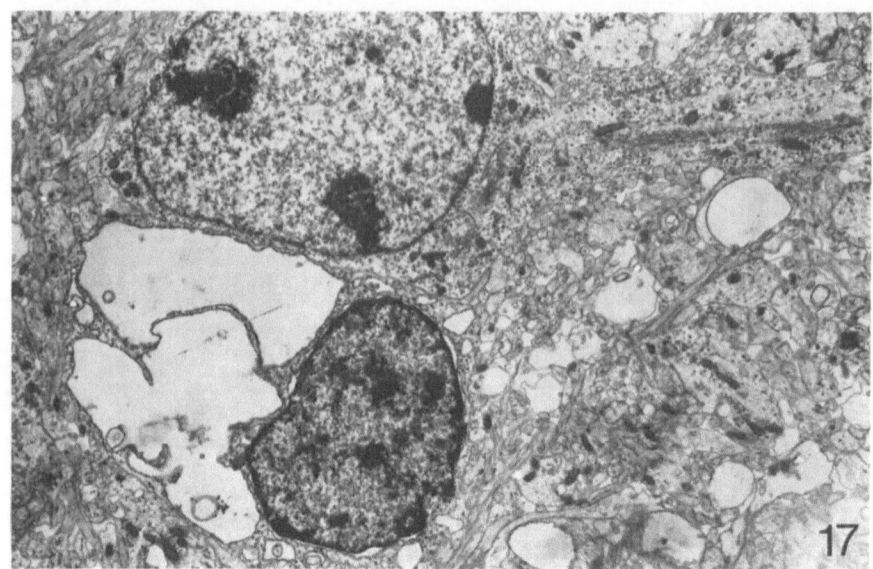

Fig. 17. Cells in the occipital neocortex of the rat seven days after birth and treatment with 6-AN. Both the perinuclear cleft and the endoplasmic reticulum of the glioblast are markedly distended. The preneuron in the upper part of the photograph is undamaged.
× 6000

Ultrastructurally the preneurons are not or only slightly damaged, some of them exhibit a minimally dilatated ergastoplasm or a modestly detached outer nuclear membrane, especially near severely damaged glia cell precursors. The perinuclear cistern of the glioblasts usually is maximally swollen, between nucleus and outer nuclear membrane thin lamellae of cytoplasm are often seen which possibly retain continuity with the rest of the cytoplasm. In the neuropil the marked distension of electron lucent processes that cannot be unambiguously identified as either dendrites or glioblastic processes, becomes noticeable. In some of these swollen processes an axon with a corresponding mesaxon were observed.

Besides these altered glioblasts that exhibit not only dilatations of the membrane systems but also a lightening of the cytoplasm, undamaged glioblasts are seen in the neuropil.

Sacrifice on the Seventh Postnatal Day

Cortex cerebralis. The vacuolar alterations of the neuropil and the glioblastic perikarya have progressed further (Fig. 17), the vacuoles are often multivesicular. Affected most is the layer directly beneath the bipolar cortical plate while the marginal zone is relatively undamaged and of normal width. All other layers are remarkably hypoplastic compared to control animals and irregularly structured. The only clearly distinguishable layers are the marginal zone and the bipolar cortical plate. The glia chambers of Held have opened at many more vessels (Fig. 16). In the white matter a few compact bundles of axons are situated directly beneath the deepest layer of the cortical grey. A little further inside, however, only solitary fibers pass through the enlarging empty space between

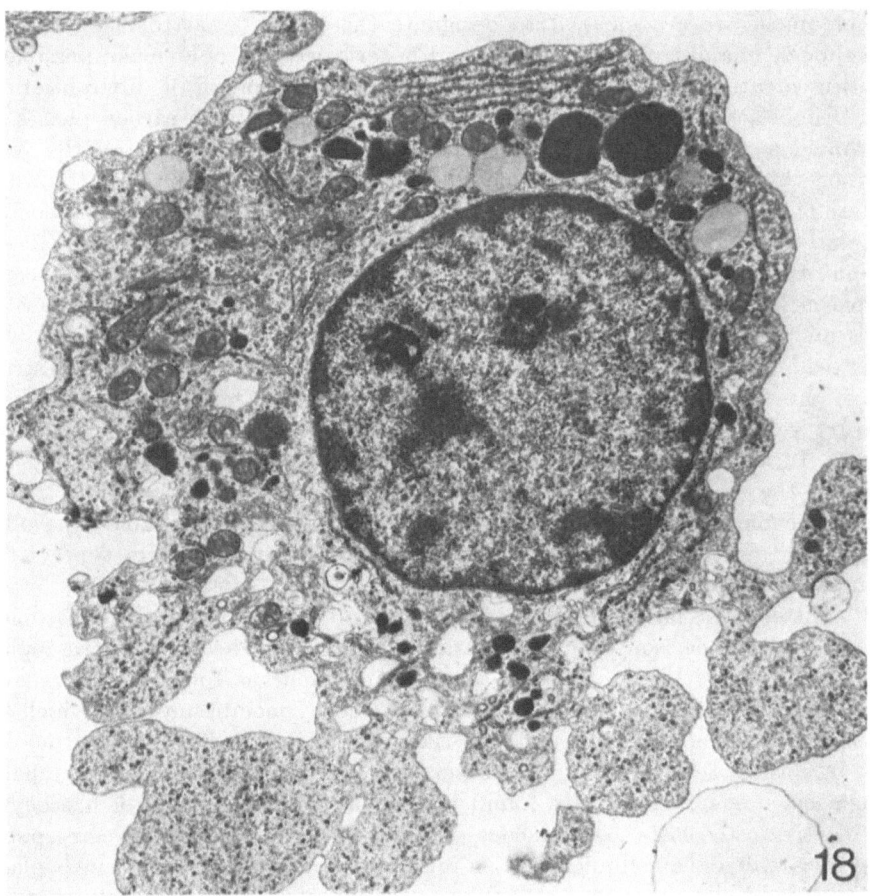

Fig. 18. Reactive cell in the cerebral medulla of the occipital cortex of the rat seven days after birth and application of 6-AN. The space surrounding this cell is empty, traversed by a few solitary fibers only, to some of which the cell is connected through its processes. × 12000

cortical grey and hippocampus, contacting scattered gitter cells and numerous other macrophages (Figs. 19, 20).

Electron microscopically, hydropic processes are seen in the cortical neuropil that are delimited partly by only membranes, partly by thin cytoplasmic lamellae containing some widely spaced ribosomes. Many of these swollen processes are not clearly distinguishable as either glioblastic processes or dendrites. The axonal fibers in the white matter appear to be loosened within the individual bundles, yet ultrastructurally they are intact as the axons in the neuropil. The different cells in the white matter can be subdivided into a number of classes:

1. Glioblasts that resemble those in the grey matter and exhibit severely distended perinuclear cisterns and correspondingly dilatated profiles of endoplasmic reticulum. These cells are encountered not so often in the white matter of the cerebral cortex. Considering the relation of their processes to the blood vessels, which in some cases are recognizable even in ultrathin sections, and the structure

of their nuclei we are inclined to designate these cells as astroblasts (Fig. 15) even though unambiguous ultrastructural criteria which would make possible a doubtless identification are not to be expected in this phase of differentiation.

2. Glioblasts that are demonstrable very numerously in earlier phases of development, and that now have rounded off their cell bodies and the perikarya of which seem to be lying isolatedly in the extracellular space of the white matter. Their nuclei have the structure of typical glioblastic nuclei with coarse, yet relatively uniformly distributed clumps of chromatin and a moderate accentuation of the nuclear margin, and overall they appear quite dark. The scarce cytoplasm likewise is relatively electron dense and with its numerous free ribosomes and ribosomal rosettes has a rather immature appearance. Besides well preserved mitochondria and granular endoplasmic reticulum the pronounced structure of the Golgi complex is especially noticeable. The few processes of these cells are relatively thin and are in contact with other cells or touch fiber bundles. In some cases the perikarya of these cells are directly contacting the axons in the fiber bundles. A few of these cells appear necrobiotic, others exhibit vacuoles in their cytoplasm which sometimes are identifiable as swollen endoplasmic reticulum, mostly cannot be associated with a certain type of cell organelle, however.

3. "Gitter cells" have been termed as such on the basis of light microscopical findings and comparison with the literature (Fig. 20). The light microscopical impression of a "gitter" (reticulum) arises from numerous round, oval or irregularly delimited vacuoles which are sharply bound by membranes, and which are so numerous in the periphery of the perikaryon that they often are surrounded by a uniformly thin seam of cytoplasm only. Similar optically empty spaces though less numerous, are also found in the marginal cytoplasm of histiocytes and inactive osteoclasts. The nucleus of these cells in its structure corresponds to a typical microglia cell nucleus with relatively homogeneous light nucleoplasm and extremely electron dense sharply contoured clumps of chromatin that are situated both in the middle and at the margin of the nucleus, usually separated from each other. Within their cytoplasm homogeneous lysosomes of intermediate electron density are observed which resemble those in the von Kupffer cells and the alveolar phagocytes, in addition to long, tortuous profiles of granular endoplasmic reticulum, lipid droplets that are not quite as sharply delimited as the vacuoles described above, and almost always round with a medium light very homogeneous content, numerous mitochondria, and sharply delimited very electron dense inclusions of various shapes and sizes.

These characteristics with the exception of the "gitter" do not occur constantly and in uniform number and distinction in all cells of this category. If the dark inclusions predominate and if these are correspondingly large we designate these cells as

4. macrophages. Within the cytoplasm of these phagocytes the electron dense, sharply delimited, sometimes irregularly shaped yet mostly round inclusions reach

Fig. 19. Occipital cortex of the rat seven days after birth and application of 6-AN. The section from the cerebral medulla shows a glioblast that is connected to fibers with its processes and that exhibits a slight swelling of the perinuclear cleft, besides a macrophage and diverse fiber sections. × 3000

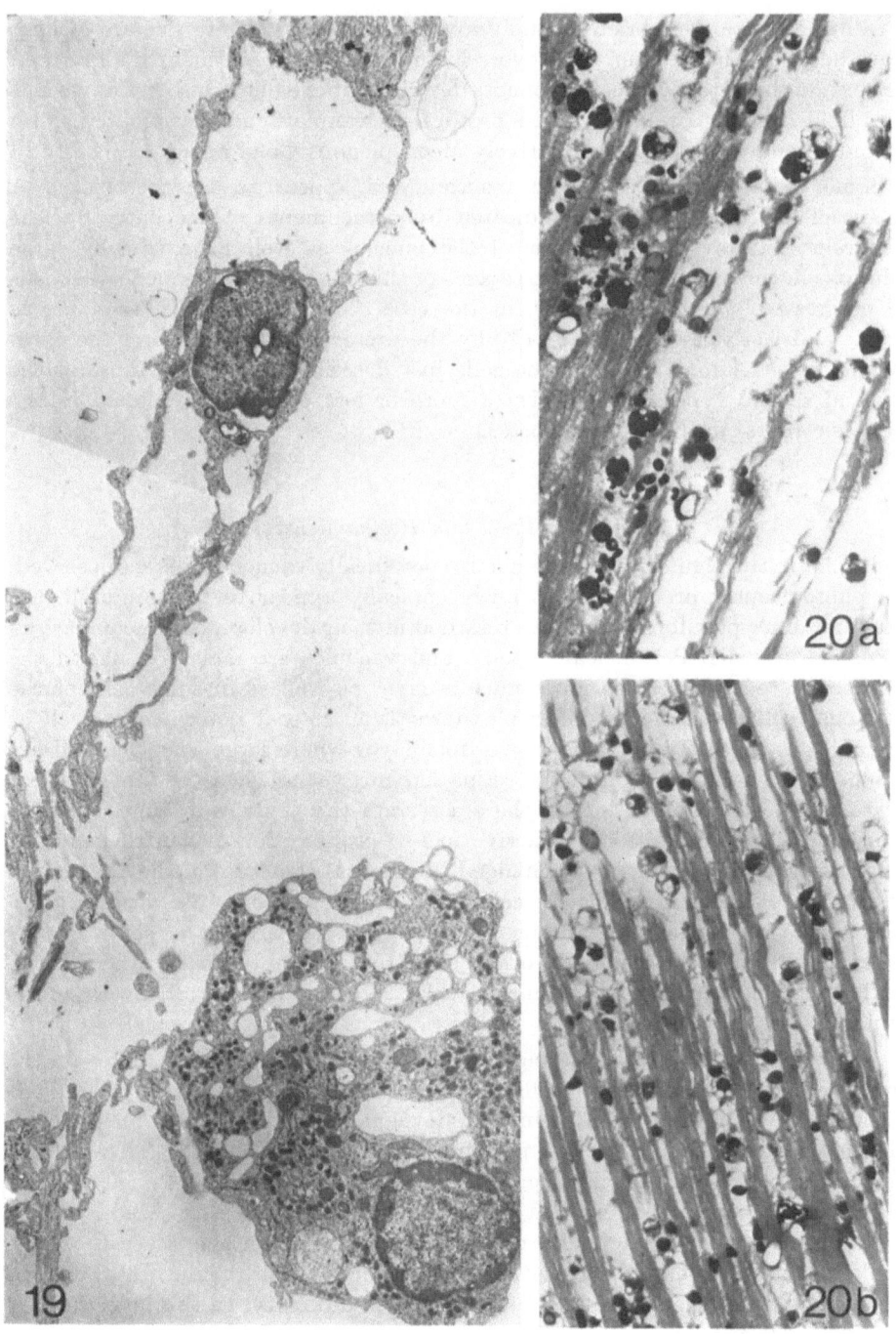

Figs. 20a and b. Occipital cortex of the rat seven days after birth (same experimental group as in Fig. 19). Cerebral medulla directly beneath the cerebral grey. Between the rarefied axonal fibers that are closely associated with glioblasts and macrophages, the extracellular spaces have enlarged further. × 192 up to nuclear size. Membrane-bound empty vacuoles of definite size are lacking or are negligible in number. Moreover, these cells exhibit a similarly structured nucleus and the cytoplasmic components described above like lysosomes of various sizes, lipid droplets, well developed profiles of granular endoplasmic reticulum and mitochondria as well as a relatively inconspicuous Golgi apparatus (Fig. 18).

Some of the gitter cells and macrophages appear to be necrobiotic. A process of cell degeneration is indicated by detachments of the outer nuclear membrane, karyolysis or pyknosis of the nucleus as well as extremely large inclusions in the cytoplasm. In later stages of this degenerative sequence the cells are progressively homogenized or, in the case of the gitter cells, the nucleus shrinks and lastly is surrounded only by the preserved membranes of the cytoplasmic gitter. A major part of the cells just described, especially those of the first and second type seem to form a more or less complete reticulum in the fiberless cerebral medulla of the cortex.

Sacrifice on the Tenth Postnatal Day

Retina. In the pigment epithelium only sporadically vacuolar cells are observed. The photoreceptor processes light microscopically appear to be uninjured, the outer and inner plexiform layers are retarded in their development in comparison to control animals. Perinuclear cisterns and vacuoles are mainly found in the undifferentiated cells of the inner nuclear layer as well as in some cells of the additional cell layer in the inner plexiform layer. Focal petechiae as well as macrophages are limited to the nerve fiber layer where large vacuoles still are present. The vascularization of the retina has not yet reached the inner nuclear layer as in normal animals. Near the ora serrata the ventricular zone is totally disintegrated, accompanied by reactive foci of proliferation of ventricular cells. These reparative processes have changed the normal structure of the ventricular zone: the proliferating ventricular cells are not anymore oriented vertically between the two limiting membranes, but fountain-like around a point on the external limiting membrane; in other sites they seem to form retinal folds. In this region a number of pyknoses still is recognizable in all layers of the retina.

Electron microscopically the pigment epithelium appears intact, likewise the structure of the photoreceptor cells the processes of which, especially the outer segments, are somewhat retarded in their development. In the inner nuclear layer undifferentiated cells with large perinuclear cisterns lie besides differentiated horizontal and amacrine cells (Fig. 21). A portion of them is sectioned without their corresponding nuclei so that they have the form of nucleus-sized, bizarrly delimited spaces without definable relationship. In the nerve fiber layer, too, large swollen chambers that are situated between intact fibers and cells can be associated with other known structures only with difficulty. In this layer solitary microglia cells are seen.

Fig. 21. Cells of the inner nuclear layer of the retina ten days after birth and treatment with 6-AN. Marked dilatations of the perinuclear clefts in the form of perinuclear cisterns that often are larger than the flattened nuclei. Many of the optically empty spaces cannot be

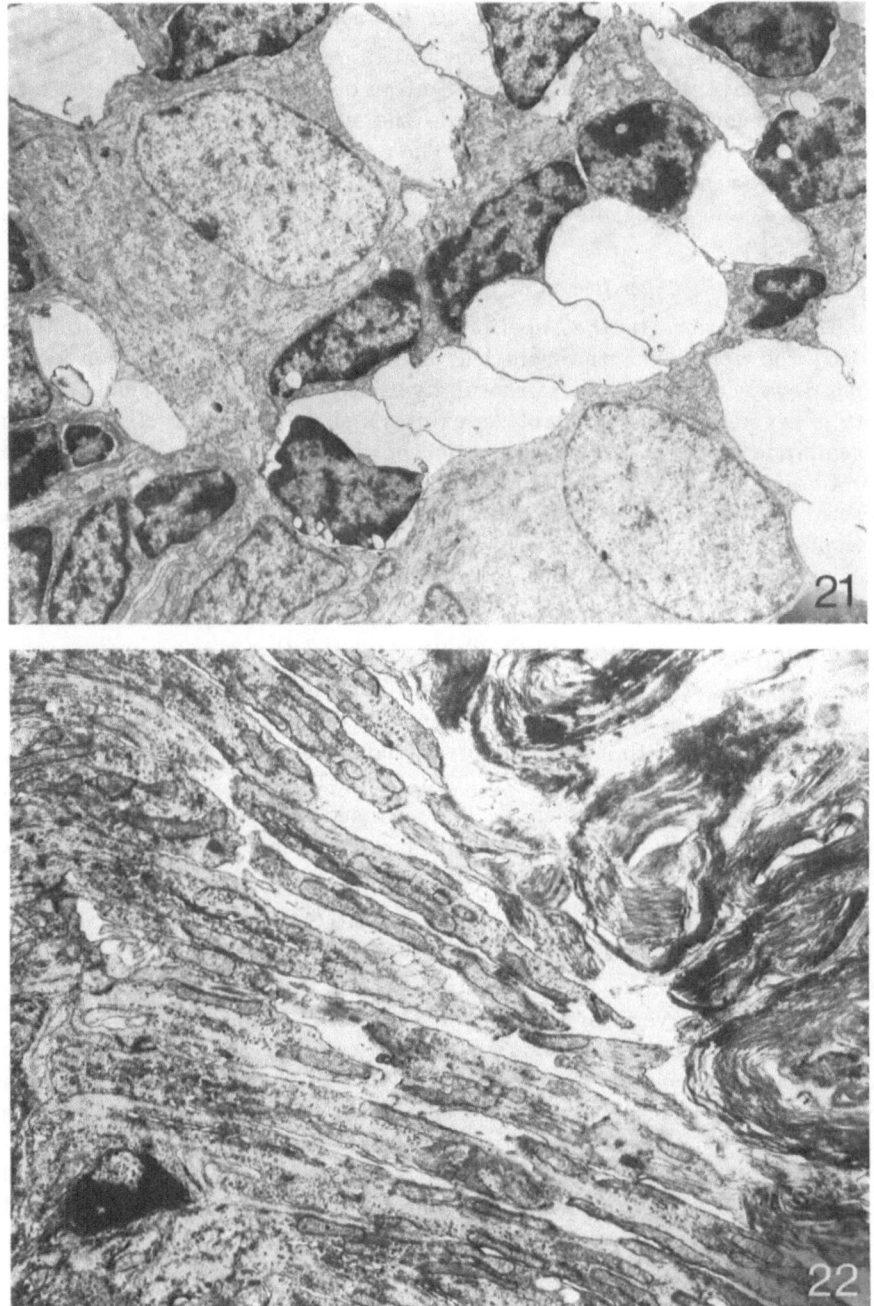

associated with a nucleus, presumably because of their size. Often the cell membranes and the thinly drawn out cytoplasmic lamellae are ruptured. The more differentiated cells in the inner nuclear layer, the amacrine cells at the border towards the inner plexiform layers, (Fig. 21) are not affected by the hydropic alterations. × 5000

Fig. 22. Photoreceptor processes of the rat retina (same experimental group as in the preceding figs.). Note the rarefaction of the processes, the shortening of their inner segments, the large intercellular spaces between them, and the concentrically coiled outer segments. × 7000

Sacrifice on the Tenth Postnatal Day

Corpus geniculatum laterale. The cytological alterations especially those in the subpial region have regressed further, so that an opposite gradient directed from the subpial basement membrane towards the ventricle is established for the regression of the pathological alterations. The cerebral peduncles are still heavily vacuolized and even more attenuated. Electron microscopically the same changes in the glioblasts and young glia cells are observed that have been described above.

Sacrifice on the Tenth Postnatal Day

Colliculus superior. In the superior colliculus the alterations have not yet regressed; the zone near the ventricle and the median proliferation center remain especially damaged. Ultrastructurally some preneurons, particularly in the vicinity of severely damaged glioblasts exhibit a slight dilatation of indeterminable membrane-bound profiles; they are not, however, retarded in their cytological differentiation. Astroblasts display detachments of the outer nuclear membrane of any size. The swollen structures often have a multivesicular structure indicating a three-dimensional structure of these damaged cells that is formed by the nucleus and some connected spherical bulbs of detached outer nuclear membrane.

Sacrifice on the Tenth Postnatal Day

Cortex cerebralis. The cerebral cortex has become further differentiated cytologically, the vacuolar changes have regressed. The histological differentiation is not comparable to that of control animals because the markedly hypoplastic cortices of the 6-AN-treated animals are not clearly laminated (Fig. 26). The situation in the cerebral medulla is unchanged. Between the widely spaced axonal fiber bundles lie numerous gitter cells. Other macrophages and pyknoses on the other hand have become very rare.

Sacrifice on the Fourteenth Postnatal Day

Retina. In the retina a general attenuation of all layers, particularly the inner and outer nuclear layers and the inner plexiform layer is recognizable. The additional cell layer has spread out further and can only be demonstrated as an accumulation of some cell groups in the middle of the inner plexiform layer, which are separated by intervals of the inner plexiform layer without an additional cell layer. Vacuolar alterations are sporadically seen in the inner nuclear, the ganglion cell and the nerve fiber layers. The retinal vascularization has reached the outer plexiform layer. Electron microscopically a rarefaction of the

Fig. 23. Inner nuclear layer of the rat retina 14 days after birth and treatment with 6-AN. The large, optically empty spaces in the inner parts of this layer mostly have direct contact with the Müller cell perikarya. Possibly they are situated directly within their cytoplasm. Besides a few amacrine and bipolar cells are seen. × 5000

Fig. 24. Section of the lateral geniculate body of the rat 14 days after birth (treatment with 6-AN on the fifth postnatal day). Opening of the glia chambers of Held, swelling of the perinuclear cistern of an undifferentiated cell lying perivascularly (upper right), dilatation of the cytoplasmic membrane systems of a glia cell (lower margin of the photograph), and discrete enlargements of the perinuclear spaces are seen. × 480

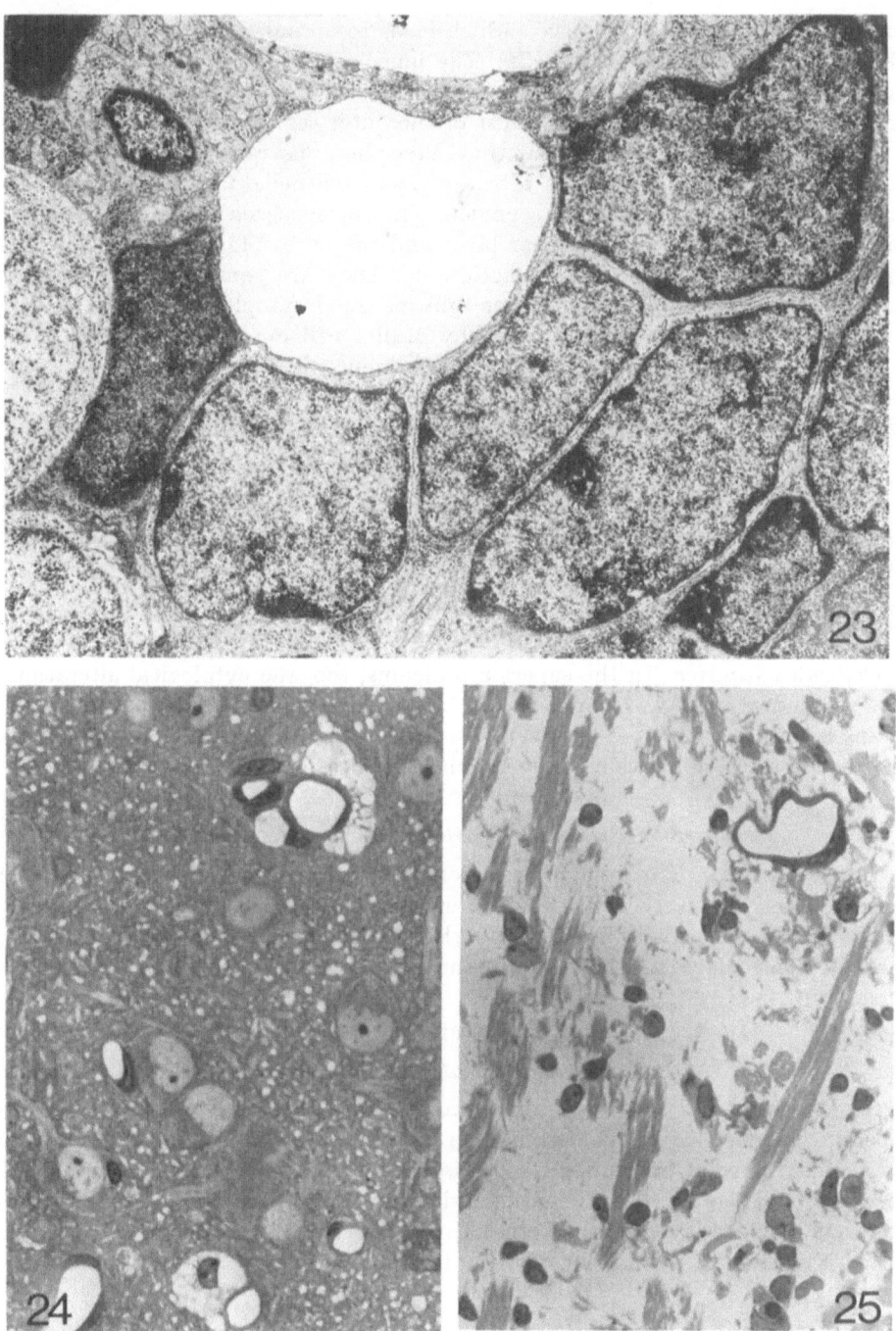

Fig. 25. Occipital cortex of the rat 14 days after birth (injection of 6-AN on the second postnatal day). Disintegrated cerebral medulla with transversely and obliquely cut axonal fibers, some glioblasts and macrophages, specifically gitter cells. The blood vessel (upper right) is contacted by a number of processes, partly, however, it seems to border directly on the extracellular space. × 480

photoreceptor processes is observed which leads to an enlargement of the extra-cellular space between them (Fig. 22). The inner segments are shortened, sometimes the desmosomal connection between them is lacking, and they contain remarkable amounts of filaments. Most of the outer segments are not elongated but concentrically coiled up so that they have the appearance of tightly wound membranes. The apical processes of the pigment epithelial cells are directed in bundles towards these coiled outer segments. The nucleus-sized chambers that have been described for the inner nuclear layer and the outer plexiform layer on the tenth postnatal day, also are still noticeable. They are generally delimited by one or two membranes and sometimes thin marginal cytoplasm adjacent to the latter. These vacuoles are surrounded by Müller cell cytoplasm (Fig. 23). The axons in the nerve fiber layer are intact, the neuropil in both plexiform layers has a normal appearance.

Sacrifice on the Fourteenth Postnatal Day

Corpus geniculatum laterale. The light microscopically visible alterations have vanished. The cerebral peduncles are markedly diminished in thickness, the vacuolar damage has regressed.

Sacrifice on the Fourteenth Postnatal Day

Colliculus superior. In the superior colliculus, too, the cytological alterations have receded even at the ventricle and in the median proliferation center. This finding is confirmed by the electron microscopic investigation which demonstrates a regression of the dilatation of the glioblastic processes and perikarya.

Sacrifice on the Fourteenth Postnatal Day

Cortex cerebralis. The cellular alterations, as in the superior colliculi and lateral geniculate body have receded. The situation in the cerebral medulla is unchanged. The cerebral cortex is very hypoplastic, a histological lamination not recognizable; only the molecular zone has reached nearly normal structure and dimensions.

Treatment on Postnatal Days 3, 5, 7, and 10

Sacrifice on Postnatal Day 14

The edematous alterations in the retina, the lateral geniculate body, colliculus superior, and the grey of the occipital cortex correspond to the findings observed in animals treated at birth after analogous intervals between treatment with 6-AN and sacrifice (Figs. 24, 25). Remarkable is a remaining sensibility of the cells of the inner nuclear layer in the retina. In the cerebral medulla of the occipital cortex a decreasing sensitiveness to the toxic agent can be related with the age

Fig. 26. Photographic montage of a cross section through the occipital cortex of the rat ten days after birth and treatment with 6-AN. The spongy alterations of the cerebral grey have regressed. The cytological differentiation has progressed. A histological differentiation in the form of a regular lamination is hardly demonstrable. The situation in the cerebral medulla has not changed, the number of undamaged fibers is especially small in the lateral part of the cortex shown in this photograph. × 110

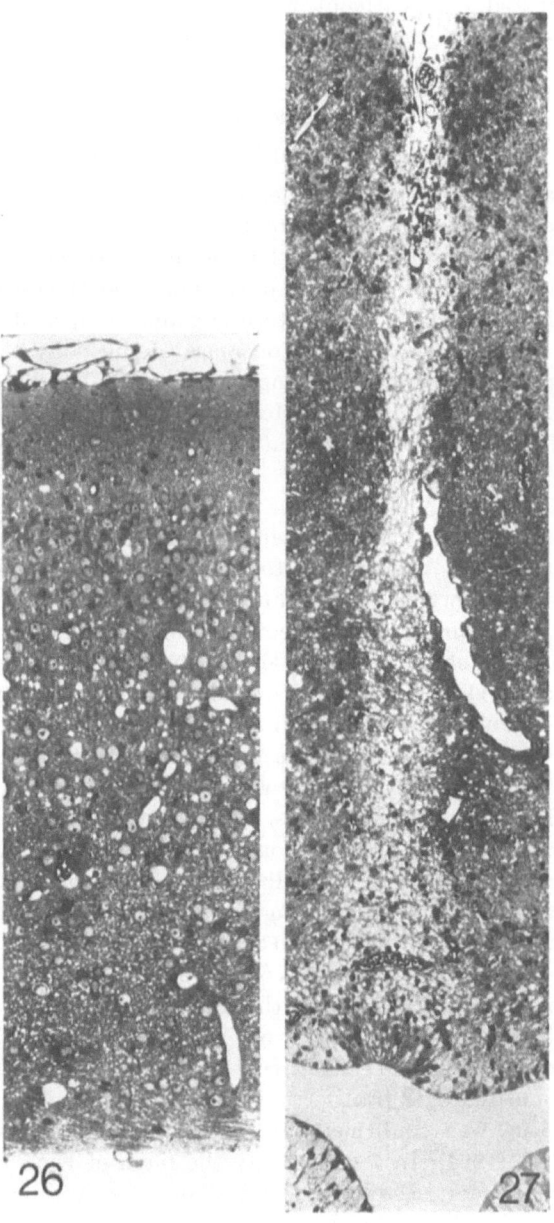

Fig. 27. Photographic montage of a frontal section of the rat superior colliculi five days after birth and application of 6-AN. Edematous alterations of the colliculus in the form of peri-nuclear cisterns of the glioblasts and dilatation of their processes at the vessels (opening of the glia chambers of Held). According to the gradient of damage that decreases from inside-out the superficial layers are affected least. A severe spongy alteration on the other hand is found in the cells at the ventricle that sometimes results in the disintegration of the tissue. To the same extent the cells of the collicular proliferation at the dorsal edge of the aquaeductus mesencephali and their fibers that ascend towards the pial surface are edematously altered. × 110

of the animals at the time of intoxication. Thus the attenuation of the axonal fibers could be effected by treatment with 6-AN until the second day of life only. Later the fibers in the cerebral medulla remained intact.

Discussion

1. Mechanism of Action of 6-aminonicotinamide

6-aminonicotinamide (6-AN), an antimetabolite of nicotinamide has been used in experimental medicine under two different aspects:

a) as antimetabolite that after administration in experimental animals results in well-defined and reproducable disorders of the brain like spastic paralysis of the extremities (Johnson and McColl, 1955; Sternberg and Philips, 1957; Wolf, Cowen and Geller, 1959) as well as a continual decrease of the body temperature and prolongation of the sleeping period following a hexobarbital anaesthesia (Redetzki and Alvarez-O'Bourke, 1962; Coper and Herken, 1963; Coper, Hadass and Lison, 1966; Lison, 1970) and leads to the formation of brain edema (Schneider, 1970; Schochet, 1970; Meyer-König, 1973);

b) as teratogenic agent.

It will be attempted to summarily demonstrate how the elucidation of the mechanism of action of 6-AN has led to an explanation of the neurological disorders of the central nervous system and the concomitant histological alterations following application of 6-aminonicotinamide.

The experiments of Johnson and McColl (1955) with the drug 6-AN, which after injection in rats led to the loss of control over the hind legs, were viewed under the aspects of antimetabolism with consideration of the study of Kaplan et al. (1954). The authors suggested that the toxicity of 6-AN depends on the formation of an inactive analogue of NAD which in turn leads to a decrease of the concentration of NAD in certain tissues. The longterm effects of 6-AN were explained by the postulate that the formation of the inactive analogue is irreversible and the tissues are not capable of catabolizing and excreting the antimetabolite. This hypothesis was soon confirmed through experiments performed by the team of Dietrich et al. (1958 a). They were able to demonstrate that 6-AN is incorporated into the amino analogues of NAD and NADP both in vitro and in vivo, which then are not capable of carrying out the function as coenzymes of certain oxidoreductases attributed to the normal pyridinnucleotides and lastly lead to an abnormal cellular metabolism and cell destruction. Moreover, these 6-AN analogues are inhibitors for some hydrogen transferring reactions and in vitro inhibit a number of phosphokinases as was confirmed later by Brunnemann et al. (1964) and v. Bruchhausen et al. (1964). In a later study the team of Dietrich et al. (1958 b) specified its formerly general assertions: not all enzyme systems depending on a certain metabolite are inhibited by the corresponding antimetabolite to the same extent; furthermore the dosis of the substance applicated determines to a great degree whether a certain system is damaged or not.

Sternberg and Philips (1957) in histological investigations attempted to associate the neurological symptoms like loss of motor control, paralyses and anorexia with well defined damaged brain regions. In their studies on rats, cats, and dogs they found marked focal destruction of anterior horn cells in the spinal cord as well as of neurons in various nuclei of the brain stem. These lesions appeared already 24 hours after application of the pharmacon firstly as petechial hemorrhages and early degenerative alterations of the neurons and progressed until their maximal development on the fourth day p.i., when they were characterized by progressive necroses and destruction of damaged nerve cells.

Wolf, Cowen, and Geller (1962), Schotland, Cowen, Geller and Wolf (1965) and Geller, Cowen, and Wolf (1966) found similar lesions and temporal pathological sequences of reaction after intoxication with 6-AN not only in the spinal cord of mice but also in numerous nuclei of the medulla oblongata, pons, mesencephalon and the roof nuclei of the cerebellum, moreover local lesions in both corpora geniculata, in the thalamus and the striatum.

In the early 1960ies a team of pharmacologists at the Free University of Berlin started with a systematic investigation of the pharmacological action of 6-AN. Like Radetzki and Alvarez-O'Bourke (1962), Brunnemann and Coper (1963a) confirmed the findings of Dietrich *et al.* (1958a, b) and found a decrease of the concentration of NADP in the brains of 6-AN-treated rats and mice. At the same time these authors (Brunnemann and Coper, 1963b) studied the distribution of the NAD- and NADP-dependent-enzymes in different regions of the rat brain in order to clarify the regional differences of reaction to the application of antimetabolites. In further studies (Brunnemann, Coper, and Neubert, 1964; Coper and Neubert, 1964a, 1964b) the mechanism of interference of 6-AN by inhibition was found to be restricted to NADP-dependent enzymatic reactions only. Finally, in 1969, Lange and Herken found the enzyme that is inhibited by 6-AN much more selectively than others since as the key enzyme of the pentose-phosphate-shunt it is present in already lesser concentrations, and in 1970 Lange, Kolbe, Keller and Herken summarized the results of the preceding studies: 6-ANADP, that has been formed in an exchange reaction betwee 6-AN and NADP catalyzed by an unspecific NAD(P)-glycohydrolase in the endoplasmic reticulum (Zatman *et al.*, 1954) inhibits the 6-phosphogluconate: NADP oxidoreductase and thus leads to a heavy intracellular accumulation of 6-phosphogluconate. The increase of concentration of this substrate in turn prevents the glucosephosphateisomerase from adjusting the normal equilibrium between glucose-6-phosphate and fructose-6-phosphate and therefore seems to be responsible for the succeeding alterations in the carbohydrate metabolism like a slowing down of glycolysis.

Almost simultaneously with the progress in the elucidation of the mechanism of the pharmacologic action of 6-AN a specification of the formerly vaguely described histological alterations ensued. In a light microscopical investigation of the spastic pareses of the extremities appearing after treatment with 6-AN, Schneider and Coper (1968) observed constant morphological damages in the reticular grey of the spinal cord (laminae VI–VIII) and in the formatio reticularis of the lower brain stem, particularly the partial destruction of the interneurons and a resulting deafferentiation of the alpha-motor neurons. Electron microscopically (Schneider, 1970; Schochet, 1970) dilatations of the endoplasmic reticulum both in neuronal and in astrocytic and oligodendrocytic perikarya and hydropic astroglial processes were demonstrated as the morphological substrate of the brain edema following the application of 6-AN in many parts of the brain, furthermore intramyelinal vacuoles as well as distensions of naked and myelinated axons with accumulations of mitochondria in the subcortical grey, particularly in the anterior horns of the spinal cord, certain brain stem nuclei and the roof nuclei of the cerebellum were observed.

The teratogenic activity of 6-AN has been described in numerous studies (Murphy *et al.*, 1957; Landauer, 1957; Pinsky and Fraser, 1959, 1960; Chamberlain and Nelson, 1963a, 1963b; Chamberlain, 1966, 1967; Turbow and Chamberlain, 1968; Barrach and Köhler, 1970; Merker and Novak, 1970; Merker, Novak and Zimmermann, 1970; Kaplan, 1973; and others). The malformations caused by 6-AN are of exceedingly various nature. Most often cleft lip, cleft palate and hind limb defects (Pinsky and Fraser, 1960), malformations of the skeleton, cns, eye, urogenital tract, thyroid and thymus (Chamberlain and Nelson, 1963a, 1963b; Turbow and Chamberlain, 1968) were reported. More recent studies (Merker and Novak, 1970; Merker, Novak and Zimmermann, 1970) indicate a so-called germ layer specificity of 6-AN according to which only derivatives of the ectoderm are damaged by 6-AN. These findings are based on experiments with tissue cultures of embryonal organs and electron microscopic studies which as the morphological substrate of the 6-AN-intoxication demonstrate an edematous swelling of the endoplasmic reticulum, particularly the perinuclear space in ectodermal cells only.

These three characteristics of 6-AN, known mechanism of action, potency of formation of brain edema, and specificity of affection of the ectodermal germ layer during embryonal development and postnatal growth seem to make appropiate the use of 6-AN in the study of the problem of brain edema in immature animals as well as for an introspection into histogenetic mechanisms of brain development by its disturbance.

2. Reactions of the Ventricular Cells

a) Stage of Multiplication of Ventricular Cells

During the first stages of the brain development studied, on days 11 and 12 of gestation, the neural wall exclusively consists of undifferentiated ventricular cells which proliferate according to the mode described by Sidman *et al.* (1959), Fujita (1962, 1963, 1964, 1967) and Fujita and Fujita (1963) and mainly enlarge the area of the brain by the formation of additional ventricular cells with proliferative potency. The probable mechanism of this growth in area of the brain has been described in another study (Raedler and Sievers, 1974).

In this stage of proliferative function the ventricular cells initially exhibit a characteristic morphological reaction in response to the disturbance of their metabolism by 6-AN. Instead of an edematous swelling of the perinuclear space which later is found as the first sign of a 6-AN-intoxication (see below) we observed alterations at the desmosomal inner limiting membrane at the ventricle as well as protrusions of the cytoplasm of the inner processes of the ventricular cells beyond the desmosomes into the ventricle which could be attributed to either a hypersecretion or a disturbance of the mechanism of secretion of the ventricular cells which according to Weiss (1936) secrete a protein-containing secretion into the ventricle during early stages of embryonal development. This reaction is found in all regions of the brain, particularly distinct in the diencephalon, however, the ventricular lumen of which is almost totally filled with these accumulations of secretions.

The typical edematous alteration of the ventricular cells in the animals treated on day 10 of gestation is not seen before day 13 of pregnancy, on day 14, however, it is so pronounced that almost all ventricular cells of certain cortical areas as well as the brain stem and the retina are damaged. These alterations regress only slowly. It is interesting to note that in cortical regions that have a very thin wall, as for instance the most dorsal part of the cortex and those that are not yet vascularized, the changes described are present faintly or not at all. The reason for this lack of pathological reactions could be either that these cells still exhibit the reaction typical for the ventricular cells of earlier stages, or that the concentrations of the 6-AN-derivatives of NADP are not high enough for a disturbance of the cellular metabolism, for instance as a result of a lesser concentration of the toxic agent because of lacking vascularization, or that these cells have originated later and not been damaged. The secondary sequels of intoxication like pyknoses, macrophages and extravasation of erythrocytes in these early treated animals occur one to two days later than in animals treated later, probably because of the delayed appearance of the intracellular edema.

b) Stage of Neurogenesis

In the stage of production of preneurons which takes place in the cerebral cortex between day 13 and 20 of pregnancy (Berry and Rogers, 1965; Hicks and d'Amato, 1968) in the colliculus superior and the lateral geniculate body between days 12 and 15/16 of gestation (Delong and Sidman, 1962; Taber, 1963; Angevine, 1970) the data found in mice have been transferred to the brain development of rats according to Hackenberger and v. Kreybig, 1965) and in the retina up to the end of the first postnatal week (Sidman, 1961) the ventricular cells display a sequence of reaction after treatment of the rats with 6-AN that is typical for this phase. One day after application of 6-AN signs of hydropic degeneration are seen in the ventricular cells and the migrating undifferentiated cells in the more superficial layers of the neural wall which light microscopically impress as optically empty spaces mostly near the nucleus. Ultrastructurally it can be characterized as a swelling of the membrane system of endoplasmic reticulum which most often affects the perinuclear space between the two nuclear membranes and thus leads to the formation of a large perinuclear cistern. Often the rest of the profiles of endoplasmic reticulum in the cytoplasm also are distended, resulting in a spongy, multivesicular appearance of the perikaryon (see also Merker and Novak, 1970; Merker, Novak, and Zimmermann, 1970).

The duration of the intracellular edema varies in the different brain regions studied. In the colliculus superior and corpus geniculatum laterale it lasts three to four days, in the cerebral cortex two to three days, and in the retina up to seven or eight days. The edematous cells that are situated in zones of proliferation immediately after the intoxication, like the outer margin or the peripheral region of the retina or in the ventricular zone of the superior colliculus, the diencephalon and the cerebral cortex are later shifted into overlying layers. The following proliferative cells, for instance in the proliferation center of the retina at the ora serrata or at the outer margin of the ventricular zone do not exhibit pathological alterations. These findings could be interpreted either as a disturbance of the perikaryal migration that normally takes place in the form of the so-called elevator movement and is characteristic for the origination of the ventricular cells (Fujita, 1962, 1963, 1964, 1967), or as a difference in sensibility to a 6-AN-intoxication or in the capacity of compensating the intracellular edema between those ventricular cells that are in the phase of mitosis and those that are in premitotic or postmitotic phases.

The cerebral edema in the stage of neurogenesis is localized exclusively intracellularly. Both in the ventricular zone with its small extracellular clefts and in the other layers of the neural wall, the extracellular space of which varies according to the stage of differentiation, a significant enlargement of the extracellular space and thus an extracellular edema is not recognizable.

The immediate consequences of the partly irreversible hydropic degeneration of the ventricular cells are the appearance of pyknoses as well as gitter cells and other macrophages; the long-time consequences are the reduction and retardation of the layers arising from the proliferating ventricular cells as for instance the bipolar cortical plate and the collicular plate. The latter has been described in another study (Raedler and Sievers, 1974). Extravasations of erythrocytes after treatment with 6-AN are found at different times of application in the various brain centers studied, usually they appear if the date of injection of 6-AN coincides with the begin of vascularization in the specific brain part. The brain stem exhibits this vascular damage after treatment of the mother animals on day 12 of pregnancy, the cerebral cortex according to the thickness of its wall in correspondingly later stages, and the retina displays regional petechial hemorrhagic extravasations in the ganglion cell layer after injection of 6-AN on the day of birth. It is noticeable that in the brain stem and the cerebral cortex the damaged vessels have enlarged to form great sinusoids which often extend over the whole width of the neural wall.

As described above, the retina remains in the stage of production of preneurons up to the end of the first postnatal week and at no point during this time interval the manner of reaction to an intoxication with 6-AN changes either quantitatively or qualitatively, so that the immediately appearing edematic reaction in the form of the hydropic degeneration of the ventricular cells and later the undifferentiated presumptive photoreceptor, bipolar, Müller cells, and the immature cells of the other layers can be provoked at any postnatal stage up to the end of the first week of life.

After injection of 6-AN on the day of birth the hydropically swollen retinal cells remain in this damaged state for a prolonged time (up to seven or eight days), while after treatment on day 16 of pregnancy already three to four days later a marked regression of the pathological reaction is observed. This temporal difference in reaction could perhaps be related to the relatively rapid differentiation of the retinal cells that have arisen early in neurogenesis to ganglion cells and amacrine cells, while the ventricular cells produced later remain in their undifferentiated state for relatively long time intervals since they begin to differentiate only after formation of the outer plexiform layer about on the fifth postnatal day (Detwiler, 1932; Weidman and Kuwabara, 1968, 1969; Braekevelt and Hollenberg, 1970; Foerster, 1973; Raedler and Sievers, 1974) and thus a large number of these undifferentiated cells is damaged after injection of 6-AN during the perinatal period. The differently sized vacuoles in various retinal layers as well as the swollen primitive processes often seen during the postnatal period that almost completely fill the nerve fiber layer, also indicate a prolongation of the undifferentiated state in which the ventricular cells are stretched between both limiting membranes (refer also to Morest, 1970b).

The capacity for compensation of the embryonal brain in the stage of neurogenesis also is differently developed both temporally and regionally. In brain regions that have a fast rate of proliferation or proliferation centers the edematous alterations have regressed a few days p.i. These brain centers are hypoplastic in comparison to control animals of the same age, yet cytologically and histologically intact and, even if retarded for two or three days, the alterations have been compensated. This uniform sequence of reaction is found in the diencephalon, the colliculus superior and the occipital part of the cortex that was studied for the present report. In the retina that has been damaged early in the phase of production of preneurons the capacity for compensation is not developed to the same extent despite a high rate of mitosis, leading to the occurrence of irreversible alterations of its histological structure. According to Hicks (1955, 1968) and Hicks et al. (1959, 1961, 1962) these usually occur only after the continuity of the ventricular zone along its apical border has been destroyed. The result may be the formation of radial foci of proliferation which could play an important role in the genesis of the prenatal retinal folds, and which are also found in later postnatal stages between the seventh and tenth day of life and p.i. mainly in the periphery of the retina, near the ora serrata. In the ventricular zone of this region focal centers of proliferation consisting of ventricular cells that are not anymore oriented perpendicular to the retinal surface but radial around a point on the external limiting membrane are situated between totally disintegrated tissue. These structures have a strong resemblance to the physiological proliferation center in the superior colliculus that for the first time appears between day 16 and 17 of gestation (Raedler and Sievers, 1974).

A true formation of retinal folds was observed only in prenatal stages of development, however, never before day 18 of pregnancy. The interval between application of 6-AN and first appearance of retinal folds was variable. In the animals treated on day 12 of pregnancy the retinal folds appeared six to eight days p.i., at later dates of injection the latency period between start of intoxication and formation of folds was shortened to 24–48 hours. Histologically the folds are characterized by an attenuation of the ganglion cell layer over the ventricular zone that has a normal width, the reactive proliferative activity therefore apparently affecting the growth in area of the retina more than the growth in thickness. The ventricular cells are edematously altered, in all retinal layers pyknotic cells are seen, particularly in the almost totally disintegrated ganglion cell layer. The excessive cell necroses are almost exclusively found in animals that have been treated early in gestation, and the eyes of which display as further anomaly an enlargement of the lens relative to the retina with concomitant severe hypoplasia of the vitreous body.

Mostly callous fusions between lens and retina either without participation of hyaloid vessels or with participation of "scanty remnants of the arteria hyaloidea up to the fusion of hypertrophied envelopes of the truncus of the hyaloid artery to the retina" (Mackensen, 1953) have been made responsible for the genesis of congenital retinal folds in the literature (Wewe, 1935, 1936, 1938; Mann, 1925, 1928; v. Manen, 1944; Mackensen, 1953; Badtke, 1954). Besides these congenital folds of the retina, retinal cysts have also been described after oxygen deficiency during pregnancy (Werthemann and Reiniger, 1950) or after application of other teratogenic agents (synopsis in Tuchmann-Duplessis and Mercier-Parot, 1961; Hicks and d'Amato, 1961). After prenatal intoxication with 6-AN retinal folds have also been reported as frequent and relatively constant malformations (Chamberlain and Nelson, 1963a, b; Chamberlain, 1966, 1967; Turbow and Chamberlain, 1968) which could be produced by injection of 6-AN into pregnant rats at any time between day 10 and day 20 of gestation. This corresponds to our findings, however it has to be viewed under the aspects of highly varying latency periods between intoxication and cytological damage as well as histological alteration, for the retinal folds never appeared before day 18 of gestation regardless of the date of intoxication.

We believe that the teratogenic retinal folds differ in their mechanism of formation from the congenital folds of the retina. Contrary to the congenital folds that are mainly produced by mechanical factors—tissue fusions and consecutive traction that results in the different foldings—we see dysregulations of the proliferative activity reactive to the necroses and edema of the retina following application of 6-AN and the resulting loss of continuity of the ventricular zone in a causal relationship to the genesis of retinal folds. The presence of a critical date for the occurrence of retinal folds during the development of the eye cannot yet be explained, however, it could be viewed in connection with the proliferative activity in the retina in relation to a shift between growth of area and of thickness of the retina, or between related ectodermal and mesodermal retinal components depending on different sensitiveness against a 6-AN intoxication of the nervous and the mesodermal parts of the eye bulb. The necroses of the differentiating cells in the inner retinal layers appearing after injection of 6-AN in early stages of pregnancy presumably represent either a primary effect as a result of insufficiently developed capacity of compensation of the early retinal ventricular cells or preneurons since they are the only differentiated cells in all regions of the brain studied that undergo degeneration or a secondary effect as the consequence of insufficient nutritional supply of these cells during the brain edema.

The findings related to the sensibility against toxic substances and the capacity of compensation of the immature brain that have been reported up to this point, are standing in opposition to those of Hicks (1955, 1958) who in experiments with various toxic substances on immature brains found a higher resistance against pathological alterations of the undifferentiated ventricular cells in comparison with their products of differentiation.

c) Stage of Gliogenesis

The phase of production of glia cells in the corpus geniculatum laterale and the colliculus superior starts about day 16 of pregnancy (Delong and Sidman, 1962; Taber, 1963; Angevine, 1970; the data found in mice have been transferred to the brain development of rats according to Hackenberg and v. Kreybig, 1965), in the cerebral cortex on days 19 or 20 of gestation (Berry and Roger, 1965), in the retina on the other hand the time of genesis of the Müller cells cannot be sharply delimited. According to Sidman (1961) they originate in the first days after birth on which numerous cells of the inner nuclear layer, where the Müller cell perikarya are situated in later postnatal stages are produced or their date of birth coincides with the loss of mitotic activity of the ventricular cells in the corresponding central or peripheral regions of the retina (Raedler and Sievers, 1974).

The ventricular cells that are mitotically active in this period of gliogenesis differ markedly from the ventricular cells of the preceding phase of neurogenesis in their reaction to an intoxication with 6-AN. The reactive pathological changes of the ventricular cells active in this period in the individual brain centers are less pronounced and shortened. Other factors like for instance altered conditions of resorption in the fetal period presumably do not play an essential role since the reaction of the ventricular cells in the retina which still are in the period or production of preneurons remains unchanged. In the period of production of glioblasts a uniform mechanism of reaction is exhibited by all ventricular cells for within this period of time the same cytological reaction can always be provoked by injection of 6-AN. The exact point of the start of the phase of gliogenesis with its change in cytological sensibility cannot be determined unambiguously since the conversion of the ventricular cells from the production of preneurons to that of glioblasts does not take place abruptly: the stage of neurogenesis fades out slowly while the phase of gliogenesis has already begun.

Ultrastructurally these ventricular cells also exhibit the typical swollen perinuclear cisterns and dilatated profiles of endoplasmic reticulum, the following secondary consequences like pyknoses, macrophages, gitter cells etc., however, are only slightly demonstrable or not at all. It may be stated then, that the difference in the manner of reaction of the ventricular cells to a 6-AN-intoxication in the phases of neurogenesis and gliogenesis is much less qualitative than quantitative. It is difficult to interpret or even to explain the different behaviour of the ventricular cells in various periods of development on the basis of our findings, especially because the products of differentiation of these last cells, the glioblasts, exhibit severe cytological alterations after application of 6-AN. Apparently the presumptive glioblasts during their genesis seem to have a lesser sensibility against an intoxication with 6-AN than either the later preneurons or the later differentiating glioblast. These findings can best be interpreted if a primarily low sensibility of the presumptive glioblasts is assumed and if the changes in sensibility are seen as the consequence of functional compensation of damages of neuronal elements.

3. Reaction of the Glioblasts

The effects of 6-AN on differentiating glioblasts is much more pronounced than the rather suppressed reaction of the glia-producing ventricular cells. It differs from the reactions of the ventricular cells described above in a number of essential factors:

a) In the latency period between injection and first reaction. While the morphological alterations typical for a 6-AN-intoxication may be already observed after 24 hours in the ventricular cells, in the glioblasts only slight detachments of the outer nuclear membrane and insignificant dilatations of the endoplasmic reticulum can be demonstrated in the first 48 hours p.i.

b) In the interval between injection of 6-AN and the maximally developed cell hydrops. The maximal cytological alterations after treatment with 6-AN in almost all undifferentiated ventricular cells appear already 24 hours p.i., in the first glioblasts not until 48 hours p.i., the majority of the glioblasts develop the maximal dilatation of the perinuclear cistern and the granular endoplasmic reticulum much later, on the fifth day p.i. in the colliculus superior and on the seventh day p.i. in the lateral geniculate body and the cerebral cortex.

c) In the time that is required for the compensation of the damages. The damaged ventricular cells of the prenatal stages on the average require three to four days to overcome the damage caused by 6-AN, and compensate a large part of the secondary consequences. The glioblasts, on the other hand, remain pathologically altered for long periods of time, in the colliculus superior for instance they still exhibit characteristics of almost maximal damage on the tenth day p.i. and in other regions like the cerebral cortex they are not capable of compensating the secondary damages caused by 6-AN.

d) In the great qualitative and quantitative differences in reaction between the individual brain regions studied. While the ventricular cells of all brain regions studied exhibit a temporally and morphologically relatively constant pattern of reaction and compensation, the glioblastic changes cannot be generalized for all centers of the brain studied. The maximal alterations of the glioblasts for instance in the corpus geniculatum laterale are developed on the fifth day p.i. In the superior colliculus and the cerebral cortex on the other hand they do not appear before the seventh day p.i. and in those regions they also show a different pattern of regression.

e) In the types of irreversible secondary consequences. As has been described more extensively above in the section on the reaction of the ventricular cells, irreversible secondary consequences of the intoxication with 6-AN during prenatal stages mainly consist in a reduction of the cell number of the affected brain centers, resulting in their hypoplasia. Damage to glioblasts, on the other hand, leads to irreparable histological defects that particularly affect the development of the neuropil, the histological lamination and the axonal fibers.

f) In the structures of the edema and its pattern of distribution. The ventricular cell edema is characterized by its rapid and uniform onset, while the edema of the glioblast exhibits a slow, progressive and protracted course.

Besides the distended perinuclear cisterns and the activation of Golgi complexes in the perikarya of glioblasts, an increasing dilatation of processes is found in the neuropil which however are not always identifyable as processes of presumptive glia cells. These swollen processes often contain irregularly shaped membranes, the importance of which has already been discussed by Kidd (1965). The edematous distension of the processes of the glioblasts moreover leads to a slow opening of the glia chambers of Held at the brain vessels, which in the cerebral cortex and the brain stem begins slowly on the third day p.i. and later spreads to ever more vessels, finally leading to a marked status spongiosus as described by Ule (1968) and Adornato and Lampert (1971).

The distribution of the edematous glioblastic cells follows two gradients. One of them is directed away from the vessel into the neuropil and corresponds to the edema gradient described by Raimondi, Evans, and Mullan (1962), the other extends from the ventricle to the pial basement membrane (apical-basal-gradient). The latter gradient could arise by an irregular pattern of distribution of the glioblast in this phase of development, which are formed near the ventricle and migrate towards the pial basement membrane. Besides the regional differences in the temporal parameters of the cytological reaction that have been discussed above, specific differences in the sensibility of the glioblastic affection of the individual brain centers may be recognized. Thus the glioblasts in the grey layers of the cerebral cortex exhibit the slightest reactive alterations following treatment with 6-AN. The brain stem on the other hand is affected much more severely and of all brain centers studied, the retina is damaged most. Differences in sensibility of individual brain regions, for instance a lesser sensitiveness of the corpus geniculatum laterale, were also observed by Lampert et al. (1965) in their study on edematously altered regions of the central nervous system following a lead encephalopathy.

Analogous to the glioblastic lesions in the brain stem and cerebral cortex, in the differentiating Müller cells of the retina numerous large, in part rather vaguely delimited vacuoles are observed both near the nucleus and in the processes. Often they are concentrated in the peripheral parts of the processes, particularly in the inner parts near the basement membrane, and they displace the ganglion cell axons of the nerve fiber layer from their innermost position at the basement membrane more to the outer parts of the retina. The pattern of lesions of the Müller cells corresponds to that of the ventricular cells of the retina in earlier stages of development, an additional fact that indicates the direct differentiation of the Müller cells from the undifferentiated proliferative ventricular cells that are stretched out between both limiting membranes (see also Raedler and Sievers, 1974).

Similar alterations or reactions are exhibited by the presumptive ependymal cells of the first to third ventricles and the mesencephalic aqueduct or the rest of the ventricular and subventricular cells. Often the cells limiting the ventricle are swollen most severe of all cells of the brain region affected, with extremely large vacuoles in their cytoplasm which in size are comparable only to the vacuoles of the pigment epithelial cells. The cells of the pigment epithelium take a special position in the pathological sequence of reactions of the cells damaged by 6-AN in so far as they develop a swollen perinuclear cistern only in the very early stages of gestation, however, then exhibit a maximally swollen endoplasmic reticulum which in turn leads to a rounding off of the cells with flattening of the apical finger-like cytoplasmic processes as well as the short processes into the system of the intercellular and basal extracellular spaces. In our opinion this different manner of reaction should be viewed in connection with the amount of endoplasmic reticulum present in the cytoplasm. In the ventricular cells and the early glioblasts very little granular endoplasmic reticulum is developed in the cytoplasm and thus the perinuclear space as part of this system is distended forming the perinuclear cistern. In the pigment epithelial cells more free intracytoplasmic endoplasmic reticulum is produced early in development—in the differentiating glioblasts and ependymal cells correspondingly later—which after intoxication with 6-AN becomes dilatated, and the perinuclear space retains its normal width.

Besides these pathologically altered glioblastic elements cells are often seen that are edematous only slightly or not at all, yet hardly differ from the damaged cells in their cytoplasmic structure. They are especially numerous in the cerebral medulla of the cortex as well as in the fiber layers of the colliculus superior and the corpus geniculatum laterale, and for the most part they are found in close relation to the fiber bundles. In spite of a certain lack of unambiguous morphological criteria in these early stages of differentiation of the glioblasts we take the majority of these cells to be oligodendroblasts, which as mature cells also have been described to be damaged very little or not at all in brain edema by many authors (Scheinker, 1938; Greenfield, 1939; Gonatas et al., 1963; Raimondi et al., 1962; Wechsler et al., 1967; and others).

The cerebral cortex exhibits a great relative and probably also absolute rarefaction of its fiber layer in the cerebral medulla beginning on the second day p.i. Between disintegrating fiber bundles, edema fluid and the various cells that have been extensively described in the results of this report are situated.

Besides the phagocytic cell types undamaged oligodendroblasts are observed which with their processes seek contact among each other and often accumulate at axonal fiber bundles or with their processes contact gitter cells and other macrophages. The origin of these phagocytotic elements cannot clearly be determined with our methods. However the following possibilities of origin exist:

1. by differentiation from undifferentiated cells of the central nervous system;

2. by development of a phagocytic function of the glia present in the brain;

3. by immigration of macrophages from the blood;

4. by differentiation from local mesenchymal cells, for instance the perivascular cells of the blood vessels.

Ad 1) Gitter cells and other macrophages are found under physiological conditions already in very early stages of embryonal development, e.g. on day 13 of gestation in the still avascular retina or the lamina terminalis of the telencephalon. The possibility of differentiation of macrophages from relatively undifferentiated cells has recently been brought into discussion by a number of authors (Vaughn, 1969; Vaughn *et al.*, 1970a, b; Skoff and Vaughn, 1971; Meyer-König, 1973). According to their findings a cell type termed multipotential glia (Vaughn *et al.*, 1970a) that ultrastructurally very much resembles microglial cells (see Mori and Leblond, 1969) is provided with the capacity to differentiate into both macrophages and macroglial cells.

Ad 2) It is known that astrocytes are able to take over a phagocytotic function and in the process can incorporate parts of myelin sheaths and even whole nuclei (Vaughn and Pease, 1970; Meyer-König, 1973). Many of the reactive phagocytotic cells in the individual brain regions described above ultrastructurally exhibit morphological transitions among each other and to glioblasts and thus could be genetically related to the latter.

Ad 3) It has been experimentally shown that phagocytes migrate from the blood into the neural tissue after destruction of the blood-brain-barrier (refer to Königsmark and Sidman, 1963) where they multiplicate and differentiate in situ to form brain macrophages. In our preparations macrophages with inclusions of erythrocytes, particularly in the vicinity of petechial hemorrhages, were found in all parts of the brain studied, often early after treatment with 6-AN; moreover numerous phagocytic cells in the blood vessels and the interstitial space were observed. The probability of a hematogenic origin of these macrophages is high according to autoradiographic findings of Königsmark and Sidman (1963).

Ad 4) The adventitial mesodermal cells of the brain vessels have been considered to be the source of the microglial elements of the brain with specific phagocytotic functions by many authors since Rio del Hortega (1921, 1932) and Penfield (1924, 1932). Maxwell and Krüger (1965) after experimental irradiation of rat brains suggested that the appearance of large macrophages is dependent on and related to the perivascular reaction, that however, mesodermal elements as for instance the perivascular cells can transgress the vascular basement membrane only under conditions of destruction of tissue. Some of our ultrastructural findings seem to confirm this theory for the conditions of destruction of tissue in our experiments were given in the cerebral cortex, particularly its fiber layer, by the disintegration of the astroblastic processes at the basement membrane and a resulting partial destruction of the latter so that the mesodermal elements had the possibility to invade the neural tissue.

It can be summarized, then, that the origin of the cerebral macrophages is not yet unambiguously elucidated and because of the variousness of the factors involved will be difficult to be determined. It is very probable, however, that the population of phagocytes appearing reactively under pathological conditions are of multiple genesis (see above) and that the constituents of this population of macrophages vary according to the type of lesion.

4. Effects of 6-AN on Preneurons and Young Neurons

The undifferentiated cells in the intermediate zone—yet not in the bipolar cortical plate—of the neocortex react to the intoxication with 6-AN in the same manner as ventricular cells with dilatation of the perinuclear space, distension of the endoplasmic reticulum and lightening of the cytoplasmic matrix. The localization of these undifferentiated damaged and undamaged cells can best be explained with the following considerations: according to a concept suggested by Berry and Rogers (1965) and Morest (1970 a) which has been modified and extended by the authors of this report (Raedler and Sievers, 1974) the preneurons necessary for the growth of thickness and for the histological differentiation of the cortical wall arise by a mechanism that is characterized by the cell division of the ventricular cells which are extended with their primitive processes between both limiting membranes, directly at the ventricle, and the migration of postmitotic daughter perikarya within the outer primitive processes of the mother ventricular cells through the intermediate zone into the bipolar cortical plate. Here the daughter perikarya are extruded from the up to now common outer primitive process—possibly in reaction to a stimulus of differentiation of the underlying further differentiated preneurons or induced by the outgrowth of axonal growth cones from the primitive process (see Morest, 1970 b) and begin to differentiate.

The begin of the metabolic differentiation of the preneurons that takes place during the last phase of migration in the bipolar cortical plate thus is connected with a significant change in the reaction to intoxication with 6-AN, for the cells of the bipolar cortical plate do not show any alterations of their cytological structure. This could indicate either totally different metabolic conditions in the cytoplasm of the preneurons after completed cytoplasmic division from the ventricular cell, or the effects of a ventricular-pial gradient of the cytological sensibility to 6-AN and a ventricular-pial gradient of concentration of 6-AN, respectively, or different metabolic situations within a single cell which are operative either as different sensibilities or different capacities for compensation and thus could explain this difference of reaction.

The first morphologically identifyable stage of differentiation of the pre-neurons has been described as the stage of beginning ramification in a study on the normal development of the visual system in the rat (Raedler and Sievers, 1974). It is distinguished most of all by a polar enlargement of the cytoplasm depending on the accumulation of a few highly active Golgi complexes and larger numbers of mitochondria which presumably supply the substrates and energy needed for the synthesis of processes, besides a shifting of the coarsely clumped chromatin to a medium coarse pattern of chromatin distribution with simultaneous lightening of the karyoplasm. The polarization of the maturing preneurons is particularly noticeable in the ganglion cell layer of the retina the cytoplasm of which is directed predominantly towards the inner basement membrane from day 15 to 18 of gestation when mostly the axons of the ganglion cells are produced, while it faces the outer parts of the retina beginning on day 19 for the establishment and maintenance of the dendritic tree in the inner plexiform layer. In the differentiating preneurons after the stage of beginning ramification and the young neurons, rapidly fading, barely visible reactions to the application of 6-AN cannot be excluded which mostly have the form of slight detachments of the outer nuclear membrane or minimal dilatations of ergastoplasm. Changes of this type were observed in preneurons of the cerebral cortex and the lateral geniculate body in the first days p.i.

Still later after treatment with 6-AN pathologically altered preneurons were found mostly in the immediate vicinity of severely damaged glioblasts. For these different patterns of reaction of the functional and nutritional unit nerve cell-glia cell to the toxic agent 6-AN, differing possibilities of sensibility and compensation have to be taken into consideration: the more severe damage of the glial cell could simply be based on a higher sensitiveness of the glial cell to 6-AN, yet, it could be possible that the metabolic disturbance of the preneurons would be compensated by the glioblasts, damaging them further, and after the glial compensation became insufficient a pathological alteration of the preneurons would result.

Truly significant changes not as much of the cytological as of the histological structure of the nerve cells are secondarily following the glioblastic reactions (also refer to Long et al., 1965). Among them are the general retardation of brain development, the consecutive hypoplasia of retina and cerebral cortex, the rarefaction of the neuropil in the cortical grey, which presumably is dependent on the deficient development of the nerve cell processes because of incomplete glial participation, as well as the swelling of some processes in the neuropil which mostly can be identified as glioblastic, although often it cannot be excluded that they are dendrites. This, however, may only be assumed provided that neuronal processes may exhibit most severe pathological alterations while the perikaryon itself from which the processes originate, is uninvolved.

Further secondary consequences are the loss of the histological lamination of the cerebral cortex and the rarefaction and destruction of the cortical white matter which is based either on an insufficient formation of neuronal axons or on the degeneration of nerve fibers already present, or on both processes. The latter secondary consequence initially appears two days after injection of 6-AN on the day of birth in the neocortex as an enlargement of the interfascicular extracellular spaces and progresses up to the formation of a gigantic extracellular edema in the region of the cortical white matter which finally is traversed by only a few axonal fibers.

Since a considerable number of fibers is present in the white matter at birth, the majority of the cortical and geniculate preneurons having been produced and ramified, and since phagocytic cell elements appear between the fiber bundles after injection of 6-AN, it seems reasonable to conclude that degenerative phenomena play the major role in the attenuation of the cortical white matter. Causally, the lacking performance of their trophic function by the glioblasts could be related to the fiber degeneration. Between the attenuated fiber bundles a large extracellular edema accumulates in the cerebral medulla which in turn could be cause or sequel of the fiber alterations. The findings in the cortical grey which exclude an interstitial edema as primary cause speak against a causal relation of the edema of the cerebral medulla to the degenerative fiber alterations.

Summarily, three possibilities of causal explanation for the rarefaction of the white matter of the cerebral cortex may be stated:

1. the primary disturbance is in the preneuron itself and leads to insufficient nutrition or formation of the axons,

2. the degeneration is related to the glial cells associated with the dendrites and axons which either because of their decreased number or metabolic alterations are not capable of fulfilling their nutritive and isolating functions, and

3. the appearance of an interstitial edema of the white matter leads to the degeneration of the nerve fibers.

According to our findings the damaging of the glioblasts seems to be the most important of these three factors which could be effected both by the disturbance of the quantitative and qualitative differentiation of the whole glioblastic population, and injuring of already functioning cell. It is difficult to estimate the relation of these two possible mechanisms of disturbance of glial cells since the cells are not yet fully mature and also do not exhibit the characteristic types of reaction following edematous alterations (see also Spatz, 1921; Sumi and Hager, 1968a, b). Thus, after Seitelberger (1965) we found a defective and a regressive but not a proliferative phase of the glial reaction. The lack of specific reactions like accumulation of glycogen, gliosis and hypertrophy to a pathological irritation of the brain before the formation of myelin sheaths has already been described by Fleischhauer and Schmalbach (1968). In our study this lack of reactive glial processes could perhaps be attributed to the shortness of the postnatal period of our experiments. It is probable, however, that the damage of the glioblasts took place in an early phase of their development in which the pathological types of reaction characteristic for the mature glia cell have not yet been established.

This assumption is based on the observation of different glial reactions in the brain stem that has been damaged on the same date (day 0). In this part of the brain gliogenesis sets in earlier than in the cerebral cortex and the majority of the glioblasts at birth has differentiated so far that alterations of the axons and the neuropil after intoxication with 6-AN comparable to those in the cerebral cortex cannot be demonstrated but the brain stem resembles that of an adult animal in its manner of reaction to 6-AN (see Meyer-König, 1973). Animals treated with 6-AN later in the postnatal period also show significant differences in the cortical reaction. Thus the attenuation of fibers in the cerebral cortex can only be provoked by intoxication up to the second postnatal day; after treatment on the following days these secondary consequences do not appear anymore.

In any case, the compensation of the edematous changes of the brain after perinatal or postnatal intoxication lasts much longer than in the early phases of the ventricular cell edema. The differences existing in the sensibility or capability of compensation between individual regions of the brain are not only quantitative but in relation to irreversible damages qualitative, too. This differing manner of reaction is in accordance with the findings of Streicher, Wisniewski and Klatzo (1965) who reported that the immature brain is more resistant to edematous alterations, as well as the results of Olsson and Klatzo (1967) who demonstrated that the blood-brain-barrier begins to function in rat embryos on day of 15 gestation and the differences in pathological reaction can therefore not be attributed to differences in permeability or vulnerability of the capillaries. Whether the regional difference in sensibility to 6-AN is a fundamentally intrinsic one, e.g. based on inherent distribution of enzymes in the various parts of the central nervous system, or related to different phases of vulnerability of the individual brain centers, cannot unambiguously be clarified with our material or methods. A phase of vulnerability according to our findings may thus be defined as a phase of proliferation of the ventricular cells during the stage of neurogenesis and/or gliogenesis, in which irreversible damages of the brain can be elicited by administration of cytotoxic agents.

Summarily it can be stated that with prenatal intoxication with 6-AN a brain edema of all ventricular cells and their undifferentiated descendants could be provoked that after Klatzo (1967) can be defined as cytogenic. In perinatal and postnatal stages treatment with 6-AN produced hydropic degenerations of the glioblasts in brain stem and cerebral cortex, which in the case of the cortical grey and white matter leads to irreversible alterations with loss of function and interstitial edema of the cerebral medulla, and a total histological deformation of the cortical lamination. The retina in its reaction to the intoxication exhibited similarities to the prenatal brain stem and cortex, yet with less potency of compensating the alterations.

5. Alterations of the Histological Development of the Centers of the Visual System

a) Colliculus superior

The embryos treated with 6-AN in various prenatal stages of development exhibited a cytological reaction that was more or less pronounced according to the time of injection, a permanent alteration of the collicular lamination, however, could not be demonstrated with our experimental set-up. The superior colliculi of the treated animals were retarded in development about one or two days compared to those of control animals and overall seemed complete yet hypoplastic. The newborn rats injected with 6-AN developed a hydrops of the collicular glioblasts and young astroblasts which led to the opening of the glia chambers of Held and a spongy state as defined by Ule (1968) and Adornato and Lampert (1971) of the individual layers. Particularly affected by this reaction was the collicular proliferation center (Raedler and Sievers, 1974) which with its dorsally directed cells and fibers is situated at the dorsal edge of the rhombic aquaeductus mesencephali. Its perikarya and fibers that reach up to the median sulcus of the superior colliculi exhibit the pathological alterations typical for the intoxication with 6-AN. In the course of these fibers damaged undifferentiated perikarya are often seen.

The spongy alterations in the superior colliculi reach their maximum between the seventh and tenth day p.i. and then regress rapidly. Differentiated processes like axons and dendrites do not seem to be affected by pathological lesions. On the 14th day p.i. the superior colliculus of the treated animals is barely distinguishable from that of control animals.

b) Corpus geniculatum laterale

The pathological lesions after both prenatal and postnatal intoxication with 6-AN do not markedly differ from those in the superior colliculus. In our opinion the reason for this similarity is to be seen in the identity of the neurogenetic and gliogenetic stages of the superior colliculus and the lateral geniculate body (Delong and Sidman, 1962; Taber, 1963; Cowan et al., 1968; Angevine and Sidman, 1961; Angevine, 1970; Keyser, 1972) that decisively influence the type of the pathological alterations. Noticeable in both primary visual centers is a gradient of cytological damage the intensity of which is directed from the ventricle towards the pial basement membrane, and which could indicate either an irregular distribution of the variously far differentiated glioblasts or perhaps a higher effective concentration of 6-AN in the ventricle with an associated lower resistance of the "ventricle-brain-barrier" compared to the blood-brain-barrier.

c) Cortex occipitalis

After intoxication of the embryos in the stages of the production of ventricular cells and preneurons the reactive behaviour of the occipital cortex does not essentially differ from that of the brain stem. The resulting hypoplasia is more striking, however, because of the reduced width of the bipolar cortical plate. The date of injection at birth just falls into the period of maximal gliogenesis (Berry and Rogers, 1965; Hicks and d'Amato, 1968) and the damage to these experimental groups affects not only the glioblasts but secondarily the nerve cells and their histological development. The genesis of the interstitial edema between the attenuating fiber bundles in the cerebral medulla has been discussed above. It can be seen in the highly reduced width of the cerebral peduncles that the number of efferent fibers decreases absolutely and not just relatively. Besides the fiber degenerations the disintegration of the cortical lamination is the most important secondary damage. Both are irreversible, demonstrating clearly that the coordinated development of neuronal processes and glial cells is necessary for the regular formation of the cortical lamination.

d) Retina

The prenatal injury of the retina by application of 6-AN in almost all experimental groups results in the formation of retinal folds. These never appear before the 18th day of gestation and presumably are characterized by focal proliferative processes of compensation below an attenuating, partly necrotic ganglion cell layer. At this time it cannot be explained why the folds appear only after day 18 of gestation, it could, however, be related to a transition of the growth in the retinal area to an increased growth of thickness of the retina. A conversion of the stage of production of ventricular cells to neurogenesis or gliogenesis cannot be unambiguously demonstrated in the retina and thus the animals treated at birth cytologically react identical to those intoxicated prenatally.

Histologically, however, at least two differences exist: firstly, retinal folds are not found in animals treated at birth but only focal centers of proliferation which have arisen after destruction of the ventricular zone, and secondly a new cell layer is formed between ganglion cell layer and inner nuclear layer dividing the inner plexiform layer in its middle. For an understanding of the formation of this additional cell layer a short discussion of the mechanisms of development in the retina seems suitable.

According to a concept that has been developed with reference to findings of Berry and Rogers (1965) and Morest (1970 b) by the present authors (Raedler

4*

and Sievers, 1974) prospective preneurons migrate within the inner process of the mother ventricular cell after their last cell division at the outer border of the retina. After reaching their later retinal localization, they are extruded from the inner ventricular cell process together with an axonal growth cone. This process seems to be disturbed by the pathological reaction of the ventricular cells which respond with a distension of the membrane systems in their perikarya to the intoxication with 6-AN, and the migration of the daughter ventricular cells very likely is inhibited resulting in the formation of an additional cell layer in the middle of the inner plexiform layer.

The pigment epithelium of the retina reacts very sensitively to the intoxication with 6-AN. The dilatation of all available membrane systems—with the exception of the perinuclear space—is most impressive. The intercellular cleft processes are flattened in the same way as the apical cytoplasmic processes. The retraction of the apical processes is perhaps related to the defective development of the photo-receptor processes which are coiled up in densely packed lamellae.

6. Prospects

The pharmacon 6-AN has proved to be an agent in experimental embryology and neuropathology the mechanism of action of which is known in detail and which renders possible well reproducable experimental studies on the brain edema in adult and immature animals. The new aspect which has been shown by the study presented and which in the future should deserve more attention, is the possibility to obtain effects in other brain regions by application of 6-AN in specific fetal and perinatal stages that are comparable to those described for the cerebral cortex and the retina in this study and thus could be used to explain the dynamics of development of the brain and the glioblastic-neuronal interrelation in differentiation.

It is suggested to treat animals with 6-AN in the stages of late neurogenesis and early and late gliogenesis of the corresponding brain regions and follow the pathological reactions up to postnatal stages.

Summary

Rat fetuses between day 11 of gestation and birth and young rats between the day of birth and the fourteenth postnatal day were treated with a single dose of 6-aminonicotinamide (6-AN) (10 mg/kg body weight) and after different time intervals the resulting brain edema and the deviations from the normal development of the central nervous system were studied in different brain regions, as represented by the visual system. In the phase of production of future nerve cells (preneurons or neuroblasts) from day 11/12 to 20 of pregnancy the undifferentiated ventricular cells react to application of 6-AN by the formation of an intracellular edema, mostly in the form of severe swelling of the perinuclear cleft, 24 hours after treatment. The preneurons themselves usually are affected by these alterations only minimally or not at all. As a consequence of the distribution of the ventricular cells the brain regions studied in early stages of development are characterized by a spongy-state-like appearance of the whole neural wall, in later developmental stages of those parts of the neural wall near the ventricle, specifically the ventricular and subventricular zones.

During the stage of production of future glia cells the reaction of the ventricular cells to an intoxication with 6-AN is markedly weaker in most of the brain regions studied; in the retina, however, where this stage cannot be definitely delineated the reaction of the undifferentiated cells remains invariably severe.

The damage of the glioblasts formed and intoxicated perinatally and postnatally again is very severe, appearing with a larger latency period of approximately three days between injection of 6-AN and morphological manifestation of the lesions in the form of dilatation of the glioblastic processes and the granular endoplasmic reticulum as well as enlargement of the perinuclear clefts into so-called perinuclear cisterns.

Prenatally the edematous alterations of the corresponding cells are compensated after a period of about five days so that mostly only a more or less distinct hypoplasia of the corresponding brain centers results. An exception again is made by the retina which displays local sites of proliferation and formation of retinal folds after extensive destruction of the ventricular zone.

After postnatal application of 6-AN the different brain regions studied show even more heterogeneous consequences of the edematous alterations of the glioblasts: while in the lateral geniculate body and the superior colliculus the damages are well compensated seven to ten days p.i., a marked hypoplasia of the cerebral neocortex with indistinct lamination as well as a progressive total disintegration of the cerebral medulla by loss of axonal fibers and formation of a massive extracellular edema develops in the occipital cortex. In the retina a deformation of the photoreceptor processes is found besides the local centers of proliferation—observed prenatally also after destruction of the ventricular zone— at the periphery of the retina and a general hypoplasia of the retinal layers. Furthermore, the normal lamination of the retina is altered by the formation of an additional cell layer within the inner plexiform layer. The formation of this new cell layer is discussed in relation to the hypotheses of Berry and Rogers (1965) and Morest (1970b) about the histogenesis of neural structures.

Acknowledgements. The authors are greatly indebted to Prof. Lierse for his patience and encouraging guidance. Prof. Dr. Neubert of the Institute for Embryonal Pharmacology in Berlin had the kindness of providing the rats treated with 6-AN. Mrs. E. Raedler's untiring help in preparing the manuscript is acknowledged with greatest gratitude.

References

Abrunhosa, R.: Microperfusion fixation of embryos for ultrastructure studies. J. Ultrastruct· Res. 41, 176–188 (1972)

Adornato, B., Lampert, P.: Status spongiosus of nervous tissue. Acta neuropath. (Berl.) 19, 271–289 (1971)

Angevine, J. B.: Time of neuron origin in the diencephalon of the mouse. An autoradiographic study. J. comp. Neurol. 139, 129–188 (1970)

Angevine, J. B., Sidman, R. L.: Autoradiographic study of cell migration during histogenesis of cerebral cortex in the mouse. Nature (Lond.) 192, 766–768 (1961)

Badtke, G.: Über seltene Duplikaturenbildungen in der embryonalen Netzhaut. Beitrag zur Genese der Ablatio falciformis congenita. Albrecht v. Graefes Arch. Ophthal. 154, 155–266 (1954)

Bakay, L., Haque, I. U.: Morphological and chemical studies in cerebral edema. J. Neuropath. exp. Neurol. 23, 393–418 (1964)

Bakay, L., Lee, J. C.: Cerebral edema. Springfield, Ill.: C. C. Thomas Publ. 1965

Bakay, L., Lee, J. C.: Electron microscopy of cat brain after hypoventilation. J. Neuropath. exp. Neurol. **26**, 169–170 (1967)

Barrach, Köhler: Wirkung von 6-Aminonikotinamid (6-AN) auf den Stoffwechsel von Säugetierembryonen. Jahresbericht 69/70 SFB 29

Berry, M., Rogers, A. W.: The migration of neuroblasts in the developing cerebral cortex. J. Anat. (Lond.) **99**, 691–709 (1965)

Braekevelt, C. R., Hollenberg, M. J.: The development of the retina of the albino rat. Amer. J. Anat. **127**, 281–302 (1970a)

Braekevelt, C. R., Hollenberg, M. J.: Development of the retinal pigment epithelium, choriocapillaris and Bruch's membrane in the albino rat. Exp. Eye Res. **9**, 124–131 (1970b)

Bruchhausen, F. von: Hemmung von Phosphokinasen durch 6-Aminonicotinamid-Analoge (6-ANAD) des Nicotin-Adenin-Dinucleotids (NAD), Naunyn-Schmiedebergs Arch. exp. Path. Pharmak. **247**, 87–92 (1964)

Brunnemann, A., Coper, H.: Pharmakologische und biochemische Eigenschaften des 6-AN. Naunyn-Schmiedebergs Arch. exp. Path. Pharmak. **246**, 63–64 (1963)

Brunnemann, A., Coper, H., Neubert, D.: Die Biosynthese und Wirkung des 6-ANAD. Naunyn-Schmiedebergs Arch. exp. Path. Pharmak. **246**, 437–451 (1964)

Brunnemann, A., Neubert, D.: Die Aktivität NAD- und NADP-abhängiger Enzyme in verschiedenen Teilen des Rattengehirns. Naunyn-Schmiedebergs Arch. exp. Path. Pharmak. **246**, 493–503 (1964)

Bunge, M. B., Bunge, R. P., Pappas, G. D.: Electron microscopic demonstration of connections between glia and myelin sheaths in the developing mammalian central nervous system. J. Cell Biol. **12**, 448–453 (1962)

Caplan, I., Arnold: Effects of a nicotinamide-sensitive teratogen 6-aminonicotinamide on chick limb cells in cultures. Exp. Cell Res. **70**, 185–195 (1972)

Chamberlain, I. G.: Development of cleft palate induced by 6-aminonicotinamide late in rat gestation. Anat. Rec. **156**, 31–39 (1966)

Chamberlain, I. G.: Effects of acute vitamine replacement therapy on 6-aminonicotinamide induced cleft palate late in rat pregnancy. Proc. Soc. exp. Biol. (N.Y.) **124**, 888–890 (1967)

Chamberlain, I. G., Nelson, M. M.: Multiple congenital abnormalities in the rat resulting from acute maternal niacin deficiency during pregnancy. Proc. Soc. exp. Biol. (N.Y.) **112**, 836–840 (1963a)

Chamberlain, I. G., Nelson, M. M.: Congenital abnormalities in the rat resulting from single injections of 6-aminonicotinamide during pregnancy. J. exp. Zool. **153**, 285–299 (1963b)

Coper, H., Herken, H.: Schädigung des ZNS durch Antimetaboliten des Nikotinsäureamids. Dtsch. med. Wschr. 88, 2025–2036 (1963)

Coper, H., Neubert, D.: Effects of 6-aminonicotinamide and other NAD-analogues on the formation of NADPH and its transphosphorylation to ATP. Biochim. biophys. Acta (Amst.) **82**, 167–170 (1964a)

Coper, H., Neubert, D.: Einfluß von NADP-Analogen auf die Reaktionsgeschwindigkeit einiger NADP-bedürftigen Oxydoreduktasen. Biochim. biophys. Acta (Amst.) **89**, 23–32 (1964b)

Coper, H., Hadass, H., Lison, H.: Untersuchungen zum Mechanismus zentralnervöser Funktionsstörungen durch 6-Aminonicotinamid. Naunyn-Schmiedebergs Arch. Pharmak. exp. Path. **255**, 97–106 (1966)

Cowan, W. M., Martin, A. H., Wenger, E.: Mitotic patterns in the optic tectum of the chick during normal development and after early removal of the optic vesicle. J. exp. Zool. **169**, 71–92 (1968)

Cowen, D., Geller, L. M., Wolf, A.: Healing in the cerebral cortex of the infant rat after closed-head focal injury. J. Neuropath. exp. Neurol. **29**, 21–40 (1970)

Delong, G. R., Sidman, R. L.: Effects of eye removal at birth on histogenesis of the mouse superior colliculus: An autoradiographic analysis with tritiated thymidine. J. comp. Neurol. **118**, 205–224 (1962)

Detwiler, S. R.: Experimental observation upon the developing rat retina. J. comp. Neurol. **55**, 473–492 (1932)

Dietrich, L. S., Kaplan, L. A., Friedland, I. M., Martin, D. S.: Quantitative biochemical differences between tumor and host tissue. VI. 6-AN antagonism of DPN-dependent enzymatic systems. Cancer Res. 18, 1272–1280 (1958)

Dietrich, L. S., Kaplan, L. A., Friedland, I. M.: Pyridine nucleotide metabolism: mechanism of action of the niacin antagonist, 6-AN. J. biol. Chem. **233**, 954–968 (1958)

Fleischhauer, K., Schmalbach, K.: Vergleichende Untersuchungen über die Reaktionsweise des jugendlichen und des erwachsenen Gehirnes nach intracerebraler Injektion von Aluminiumhydroxyd. Acta neuropath. (Berl.) **11**, 311–337 (1968)

Förster, H.: Postnatale Organogenese und Zytotopographie der Retina. Acta anat. (Basel) **84**, 321–352 (1973)

Fujita, S.: Kinetics of cellular proliferation. Experim. Cell Res. **28**, 52–60 (1962)

Fujita, S.: Matrix cells and cytogenesis of the developing cns. J. comp. Neurol. **120**, 37–42 (1963)

Fujita, S.: Applications of light and electron microscopy, and autoradiography to the study of cytogenesis of the forebrain. In: Evolution of the forebrain. Ed. by R. Hassler and H. Stephan, p. 180–196. New York: Plenum Press 1967

Fujita, H., Fujita, S.: Electron microscopic observations on the histogenesis of the cns. (I) On the nerve cell differentiation. Acta anat. Nippon **38**, 85–94 (1963)

Geller, L. M., Cowen, D., Wolf, A.: Effect of the antimetabolite, 6-aminonicotinamide, on soundinduced seizures in mice. Exp. Neurol. **14**, 86–98 (1966)

Gonatas, N.: Comparative study of status spongiosus. 6. Intern. Kongr. f. Neuropath. Paris: Masson & Cie 1970

Gonatas, N., Zimmermann, H. M., Levin, S.: Ultrastructure of inflammation with edema in the rat brain. Amer. J. Path. **42**, 455–469 (1963)

Greenfield, J. G.: The history of cerebral edema associated with intracranial tumors. Brain **62**, 129–152 (1939)

Hackenberg, J., Kreybig, Th.: Vergleichende teratologische Untersuchungen bei der Maus und der Ratte. Arzneimittel-Forsch. (Drug. Res.) **15**, 1456–1460 (1965)

Herken, H.: Antimetabolic action of 6-AN on the pentose phosphate pathway in the brain. In: Alridge, W. N. (ed.), Mechanisms of toxicity, p. 189–203. London-Macmillan Co. Ltd. 1971

Herken, H., Lange, K.: Blocking of pentose phosphate pathway in the brain of rats by 6-AN. Naunyn-Schmiedebergs Arch. exp. Path. Pharmak. **263**, 496–499 (1969)

Hicks, S. P.: Effects of ionizing radiation, certain hormones and radiomimetic drugs on the developing nervous system. J. cell. comp. Physiol. **43** (Suppl.), 151–178 (1954a)

Hicks, S. P.: Mechanisms of radiation anencephaly, anophthalmia and pituitary anomalies. Repair in the mammalian embryo. Arch. Path. **57**, 1–16 (1954b)

Hicks, S. P.: Developmental brain metabolism. Effects of cortisone, anoxia, fluoroacetate, radiation, insulin, and other inhibitors on the embryo, newborn, and adult. Arch. Path. **55**, 302–327 (1955)

Hicks, S. P.: Radiation as an experimental tool in mammalian developmental neurology. Physiol. Rev. **38**, 337–356 (1958)

Hicks, S. P., Brown, B. Z., D'Amato, C. J.: Regeneration and malformation in the nervous system, eye, and mesenchyme of the mammalian embryo after radiation injury. Amer. J. Path. **33**, 459–481 (1957)

Hicks, S. P., D'Amato, C. J., Lowe, M. J.: Development of the mammalian nervous system. Malformation of the brain, especially the cerebral cortex induced in rats. J. comp. Neurol. **113**, 435–470 (1959)

Hicks, S. P., Cavanaugh, M. C., O'Brien, E. D.: Effects of anoxia on the developing cerebral cortex in the rat. Amer. J. Path. **40**, 61–63 (1962)

Hicks, S. P., D'Amato: How to design and build abnormal brains using radiation during development. In: Disorders of the developing nervous system. W. S. Fields and M. M. Desmond, eds., chap. 4, p. 60–97. Springfield, Ill. Charles C. Thomas 1961

Hicks, S. P., D'Amato, C. J.: Cell migrations to the isocortex in the rat. Anat. Rec. **160**, 619–634 (1968)

Johnson, W. J., McColl, J. D.: 6-AN—a potent nicotinamide antagonist. Science **122**, 834 (1955)

Johnson, W. J., McColl, J. D.: Antimetabolite activity of 6-AN. Fed. Proc. **15**, 284 (1956)

Keyser, A.: The development of the diencephalon of the Chinese hamster. Acta anat. (Basel), Suppl. 59 ad Vol. 83 (1972)

Kidd, M.: Ultrastructure aspects of status spongiosus. In: Brain edema, ed. by Klatzo, I./ Seitelberger, F. (1967)

Klatzo, I.: Neuropathological aspects of brain edema. J. Neuropath. exp. Neurol. **26**, 1–14 (1967)

Klatzo, I.: Some morphological and biochemical aspects of abnormal glycogen accumulation in the glia. 6. Internationaler Kongreß für Neuropathologie. Paris: Masson & Cie. 1970

Klatzo, I., Piraux, A., Laskowski, E.: The relationship between edema, blood brain barrier, and tissue elements in local brain injury. J. Neuropath. exp. Neurol. **17**, 548–563 (1958)

Koenigsmark, B. W., Sidman, R. L.: Origin of brain macrophages in the mouse. J. Neuropath. exp. Neurol. **22**, 643–676 (1963)

Lampert, P.: Electron microscopic studies on ordinary and hyperacute experimental allergic encephalomyelits. Acta neuropath. (Berl.) **9**, 99–126 (1967)

Lampert, P., Garro, F., Pentschew, A.: Lead encephalopathy in suckling rats. In: Brain edema, ed. by Klatzo, I./Seitelberger, F. (1967)

Landauer, W.: Niacin antagonists and chick development. J. exp. Zool. **136**, 509 (1957)

Lange, K., Kolbe, H., Keller, K., Herken, H.: Der Kohlenhydratstoffwechsel des Gehirns nach Blockade des Pentosephasphat-Weges durch Aminonicotinsäureamid. Hoppe-Seylers Z. physiol. Chem. **351**, 1241–1252 (1970)

Lison, H.: Untersuchungen zur Differenzierung der durch 6-Aminonicotinamid, einem Anti-metaboliten des Nicotinamids, hervorgerufenen zentralnervösen Funktionsstörungen. Naunyn-Schmiedebergs Arch. exp. Path. Pharmak. **267**, 155–169 (1960)

Luft, J. H.: Improvements in epoxy resin embedding methos. J. biophys. biochem. Cytol. **9**, 409–414 (1961)

Mackensen, G.: Angeborene Netzhautfalten und Persistenz der Glaskörpergefäße. Klin. Mbl. Augenheilk. **123**, 417–433 (1953)

Manen, J. G. van: Décollement rétinien falciforme congenital et anomalies congenitales connexes. Ophthalmologica (Basel) **107**, 121–148 (1944)

Mann, I.: A rare case of congenital abnormality of the retina. Trans. ophthal. Soc. U.K. **48**, 383 (1928)

Mann, I.: Congenital retinal fold. Brit. J. Ophthal. **19**, 641–658 (1935)

Maxwell, D. S., Kruger, L.: Small blood vessels and the origin of phagocytes in the rat cerebral cortex following heavy particle irradiation. Exp. Neurol. **12**, 33–54 (1965)

Meller, K.: Histo- und Zytogenese der sich entwickelnden Retina. Veröff. morph. Path. H 77 (1968)

Merker, H. J., Novack, L.: Störungen der Zahnentwicklung bei Rattenembryonen nach Gaben von 6-AN. Experientia (Basel) **26**, 1127 (1970)

Merker, H. J., Novack, L., Zimmermann, B.: Elektronenmikroskopische Untersuchungen über die Wirkung von 6-AN auf Säugetierembryonen. Naunyn-Schmiedebergs Arch. Pharmak. **266**, 401 (1970)

Morest, D. K.: A study of neurogenesis in the forebrain of opossum pouch young. Z. Anat. Entwickl.-Gesch. **130**, 265–305 (1970a)

Morest, D. K.: The pattern of neurogenesis in the retina of the rat. Z. Anat. Entwickl.-Gesch. **131**, 45–67 (1970b)

Mori, S., Leblond, C. P.: Identification of microglia in light and electron microscopy. J. comp. Neurol. **135**, 57–80 (1969a)

Mori, S., Leblond, C. P.: Electron microscopic features and proliferation of astrocytes in the corpus callosum of the rat. J. comp. Neurol. **137**, 197–226 (1969b)

Mugnaini, G., Walberg, F.: Ultrastructure of neuroglia. Ergebn. Anat. Entwickl.-Gesch. **37**, 194–236 (1964)

Murphy, M. L., Dagg, C. P., Karnofsky, D. A.: Comparison of teratogenic chemicals in the rat and chick embryos. Pediatrics **19**, 701–714 (1957)

Nemetschek-Gansler, H.: Zur Ultrastruktur dunkler Neurone. Erg.-Bd. Anat. Anz. **113**, 328–333 (1964)

Ofori-Nkansah, Bruchhausen, F. von: Some metabolic and morphological alterations in Yoshida ascites tumour cells caused by 6-aminonicotinamide. Z. Krebsforsch. **77**, 64–76 (1972)

Olsson, Y., Klatzo, I., Sourander, P., Steinwall, O.: Blood-brain barrier to albumin in embryonic new born and adult rats. Acta neuropath. (Berl.) **10**, 117–122 (1967)

Penfield, W.: Oligodendroglia and its relation to classical neuroglia. Brain **47**, 430–452 (1924)

Penfield, W.: Neuroglia: normal and pathological. In: Cytology and cellular pathology of the nervous system. W. Penfield, ed. New York: Hoeber 1932

Penfield, W., Buckley, R.: Punctures of the brain. Arch. Neurol. Psychiat. **20**, 1–13 (1938)

Pinsky, L., Fraser, F. C.: Congenital malformations after a two-hour inactivation of nicotin-amide in pregnant mice. Brit. med. J. 2 V, 195–197 (1960)

Pryszkowski, V., Lierse, W., Franke, H. D.: Histochemische und ultrastrukturelle Frühver-änderungen des Meerschweinchengehirns nach Bestrahlung mit 17 MeV Betastrahlen. Acta neuropath. (Berl.) **11**, 338–346 (1968)

Raimondi, A. J., Clasen, R. A., Beattie, E. J., Taylor, C. B.: The effect of hypothermia and steroid therapy on experimental cerebral injury. Surg. Gynec. Obstet. **108**, 333–338 (1959)

Raimondi, A. J., Evans, J. P., Mullan, S.: Studies of cerebral edema. III. Alterations in the white matter. Acta neuropath. (Berl.) **2**, 177–197 (1962)

Ramsey, H.: Differentiation of oligodendroglia from migratory spongioblasts. 5. Int. Cong. Electron Microsc., Philadelphia, vol. II, N-3. New York: Acad. Press 1962

Redetzki, H. M., O-Bourke, A.: 6-AN a central nervous system depressant. J. Pharmacol. exp. Ther. **137**, 173–178 (1962)

Reynolds, E. S.: The use of lead citrate at high ph as an electron opaque stain in electron microscopy. J. Cell Biol. **17**, 208–212 (1963)

Rio-Hortega, P. del: Microglia. In: Cytology and cellular pathology of the nervous system. W. Penfield, ed., Vol. II, p. 482–544. New York: Hoeber 1932

Scheinker, I.: Zur Histopathologie des Hirnödems und der Hirnschwellung bei Tumoren des Gehirns. Dtsch. Z. Nervenheilk. **147**, 137–162 (1938)

Schneider, H.: Schädigung der Formatio reticularis durch den Antimetaboliten 6-Amino-nicotinamid. VI. Internationaler Kongreß für Neuropathologie. Paris: Masson & Cie. 1970

Schneider, H., Coper, H.: Morphologische Befunde am Zentralnervensystem der Ratte nach Vergiftung mit Antimetaboliten des Nicotinamids (6-Aminonicotinsäureamid und 3-Acetylpyridin) und einem Chinolinderivat (5-Nitro-8-hydroxychinolin). Arch. Psychiat. Nervenkr. **211**, 138–154 (1968)

Schochet, S.: Pathogenesis of 6-aminonicotinamide neurotoxicity. In: VI. Internationaler Kongreß für Neuropathologie. Paris: Masson & Cie. 1970

Schotland, D. J., Cowen, D., Geller, L. M., Wolf, A.: A histochemical study of the effects of an antimetabolite, 6-AN on the spinal cord of the adult rat. J. Neuropath. exp. Neurol. **24**, 97–107 (1965)

Sidman, R. L.: Histogenesis of mouse retina studied with thymidine-H^3. In: The structure of the eye. Smelser ed., p. 487–506 New York: Academic Press 1961

Sidman, R. L.: Autoradiographic methods and principles for study of the nervous system with thymidine-H^3. In: Contemporary research methods in neuroanatomy. Ed. by Nauta, W. J. H., and Ebbesson, S. O. E. (1970)

Sidman, R. L., Miale, I. L., Feder, N.: Cell proliferation and migration in the primitive epen-dymal zone, an autoradiographic study of histogenesis in the nervous system. Exp. Neurol. **1**, 322–333 (1959)

Sievers, J.: Basic two-dye stains for epoxy-embedded 0,3-1 μ sections. Stain Technol. **46**, 196–199 (1971)

Skoff, R. P., Vaughn, J. E.: An autoradiographic study of cellular proliferation in degenerating rat optic nerve. J. comp. Neurol. **141**, 133–156 (1971)

Spatz, H.: Über die Vorgänge nach experimenteller Rückenmarksdurchtrennung mit beson-derer Berücksichtigung der Unterschiede der Reaktionsweise des reifen und des unreifen Gewebes nebst Beziehungen zur menschlichen Pathologie (Porenzephalie und Syringo-myelie). Nissel-Alzheimer Histolog. Histopath. Arb. E.B. 49–364 (1921)

Sternberg, S. S., Philips, F. S.: 6-AN and acute degenerative changes in the central nervous system. Science **127**, 644–646 (1957)

Sternberg, S. S., Philips, F. S.: Biological effects of 6-AN. Bull. N.Y. Acad. Med. **35**, 811 (1959)

Streicher, E., Wisniewski, H., Klatzo, I.: Resistance of immature brain to experimental cerebral edema. Neurology (Minneap.) **15**, 833–836 (1965)

Sumi, S. M., Hager, H.: Electron microscopic study of the reaction of the new born rat brain to injury. Acta neuropath. (Berl.) **10**, 324–335 (1968)

Sumi, S. M., Hager, H.: Electron microscopic features of an experimentally produced porencephalic cyst in the rat brain. Acta neuropath. (Berl.) **10**, 336–346 (1968)

Taber, E.: Histogenesis of brain stem neurons studied autoradiographically with thymidine-H^3 in the mouse. Anat. Rec. **145**, 291 (1963)

Tuchmann-Duplessis, H., Mercier-Parot, L.: Production of congenital eye malformations, particularly in rat fetuses. In: Structure of the eye. G. K. Smelser ed., p. 507–520. New York: Academic Press 1961

Turbow, M. M., Chamberlain, J. G.: Direct effects of 6-aminonicotinamide on the developing rat embryo in vitro and in vivo. Teratology 1, 103–108 (1968)

Ule, G.: Elektronenmikroskopische Studien zum experimentellen Hirnödem. In: IV. Internationaler Kongreß für Neuropathologie, ed. H. Jakob, vol. 2. Stuttgart: Thieme 1963

Ule, G.: Zur Ultrastruktur der Astroglia, und des Status spongiosus. Acta neuropath. (Berl.), Suppl. IV (1968)

Vaughn, J. E.: An electron microscopic analysis of gliogenesis in rat optic nerves. Z. Zellforsch. 94, 293–324 (1969)

Vaughn, J. E., Hinds, P. L., Skoff, R. P.: Electron microscopic studies of Wallerian degeneration in rat optic nerves. 1. The multipotential glia. J. comp. Neurol. 140, 175–205 (1970)

Vaughn, J. E., Pease, D. C.: Electron microscopic studies of Wallerian Degeneration in rat optic nerves. II. Astrocytes, oligodendrocytes and adventitial cells. J. comp. Neurol. 140, 207–225 (1970)

Wechsler, W., Riverson, E., Schröder, J. M., Kleihues, P., Palmeiro, J. F., Hossmann, K. A.: Electron microscopic observations on different models of acute experimental brain edema. In: Brain edema, ed. by Klatzo, I., and Seitelberger, F. Berlin-Heidelberg-New York: Springer 1967

Weed, L. H., McKibben, P. S.: Experimental alterations of brain bulk. Amer. J. Physiol. 48, 531–558 (1919)

Weidman, T. A., Kuwabara, T.: Postnatal development of the retina. Arch. Ophthal. 79, 470–484 (1968)

Weiss, P.: Secretory activity of the inner layer of the embryonic midbrain of the chick as revealed by tissue culture. Anat. Rec. 58, 299–302 (1933/34)

Werthemann, P., Reiniger, M.: Über Augenentwicklungsstörungen bei Rattenembryonen durch Sauerstoffmangel in der Frühschwangerschaft. Acta anat. (Basel) 11, 329–347 (1950)

Wewe, H.: Über Ablatio falciformis congenita. Arch. Augenheilk. 109, 49–78 (1936)

Wewe, H.: Ablatio falciformis congenita (retinal fold). Brit. J. Ophthal. 22, 456–470 (1938)

Wolf, A., Cowen, D.: Pathological changes in the central nervous system produced by 6-AN. Bull. N.Y. Acad. Med. 35, 814–817 (1959)

Wolf, A., Cowen, D., Geller, L. M.: The effects of an antimetabolite, 6-AN on the cns. Trans. Amer. neurol. Ass. 140 (1959)

Zatman, L. J., Kaplan, N. O., Colowick, S. P., Ciotti, M. M.: The isolation and properties of the isonicotinic acid hydrazide analogue of diphosphopyridine nucleotide. J. biol. Chem. 209, 467–484 (1954)

Subject Index